Operation Beautiful

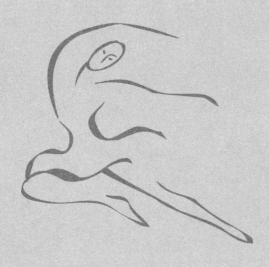

"Powerful, inspiring, and yes, beautiful: *Operation Beautiful* is the perfect gift for teens, friends, daughters, moms . . . and to ourselves."

—Julia DeVillers, author of *GirlWise: How to Be Confident, Capable, Cool, and In Control*

"This ingenious book is a refreshing take on how to help women feel empowered, beautiful, and, finally, put an end to 'Fat Talk'! It's a must-read for everyone."

—Susan Albers, author of *Eating Mindfully: How to End Mindless Eating and Enjoy a Balanced Relationship with Food*

"Finally, a counterculture movement to uplift the spirits of womankind. . . . Normally we use Post-it notes to remind ourselves of some arduous chore we need to do; yet Caitlin Boyle has shown women how to pay it forward, reminding others that they are beautiful inside and out. Carry on this revolution, ladies!"

—Denise Martz, Ph.D., professor of psychology, Appalachian State University

"*Operation Beautiful* reflects a revolution for women that is long overdue. Kudos to Caitlin Boyle for inspiring monumental change with one simple and very brave act."

—Joy Jacobs, J.D., Ph.D., clinical psychologist

"*Operation Beautiful* is an uplifting book about the power of positive thinking. Inside this small gem, we find the voices of women of all ages, shapes, and sizes who have moved away from Fat Talk to love and respect who they are. Reading their stories reminds us that we have the ability to change and feel good about ourselves each and every day!"

—Mimi Nichter, author of *Fat Talk: What Girls and Their Parents Say about Dieting*

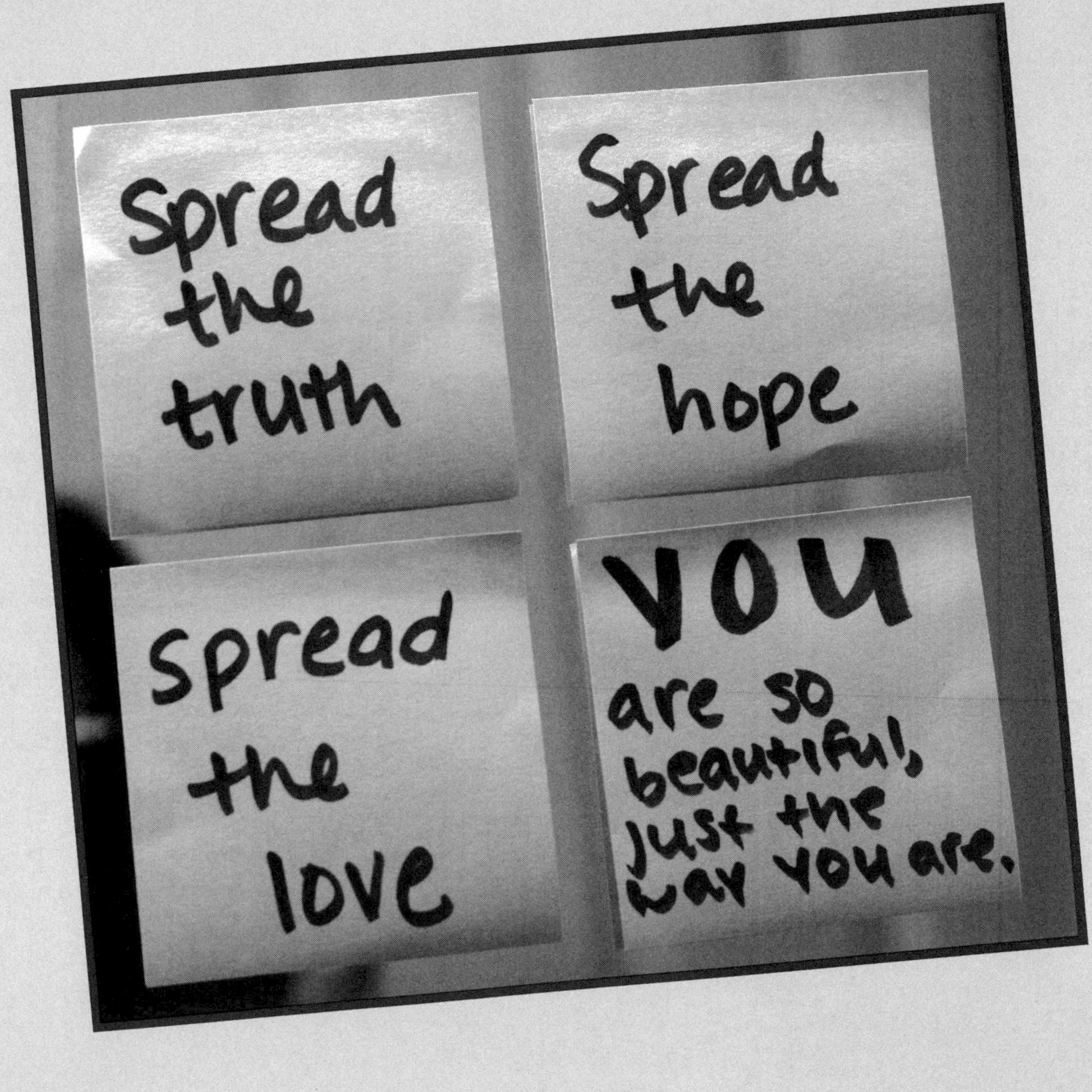
Spread the truth
Spread the hope
Spread the love
YOU are so beautiful, just the way you are.

Operation Beautiful

Transforming Yourself
One Post-it Note at a Time

Caitlin Boyle

GOTHAM
BOOKS

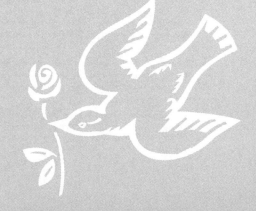

GOTHAM BOOKS
Published by Penguin Group (USA) Inc.
375 Hudson Street, New York, New York 10014, U.S.A.
Penguin Group (Canada), 90 Eglinton Avenue East, Suite 700, Toronto, Ontario M4P 2Y3, Canada (a division of
Pearson Penguin Canada Inc.) · Penguin Books Ltd, 80 Strand, London WC2R 0RL, England · Penguin Ireland, 25
St Stephen's Green, Dublin 2, Ireland (a division of Penguin Books Ltd) · Penguin Group (Australia), 250 Camberwell
Road, Camberwell, Victoria 3124, Australia (a division of Pearson Australia Group Pty Ltd) · Penguin Books India Pvt
Ltd, 11 Community Centre, Panchsheel Park, New Delhi—110 017, India · Penguin Group (NZ), 67 Apollo Drive,
Rosedale, North Shore 0632, New Zealand (a division of Pearson New Zealand Ltd) · Penguin Books (South Africa)
(Pty) Ltd, 24 Sturdee Avenue, Rosebank, Johannesburg 2196, South Africa

Penguin Books Ltd, Registered Offices: 80 Strand, London WC2R 0RL, England

Published by Gotham Books, a member of Penguin Group (USA) Inc.

First printing, August 2010
10 9 8 7 6 5 4 3 2 1

Gotham Books and the skyscraper logo are trademarks of Penguin Group (USA) Inc.

LIBRARY OF CONGRESS CATALOGING-IN-PUBLICATION DATA

Boyle, Caitlin.
    Operation beautiful : transforming yourself one post-it note at a time
/ Caitlin Boyle.
    p. cm.
    ISBN 978-1-592-40582-4 (pbk.)
    1. Body image in women. 2. Self-esteem in women. 3. Self-perception in women. I. Title.
    BF697.5.B63B69 2010
    646.70082—dc22   2010008874

Printed in the United States of America

Set in Mrs Eaves · Designed by Sabrina Bowers & Elke Sigal

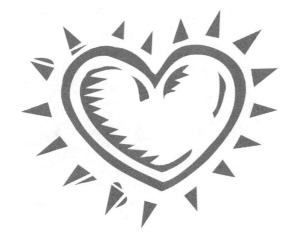

To Kristien,
Who gave me wings,

And to my parents,
Who gave me roots.

Contents

Operation Beautiful

Chapter 1

Introduction

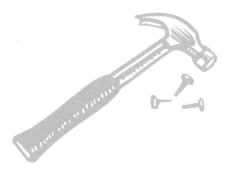

My name is Caitlin, and for many years I was my own worst enemy.

When I was thirteen years old, anger burned inside me. The heat never waned. My emotions were so volatile that I barely scraped by each day without losing it. On the outside, things seemed fine, but privately, I was suffocating under the weight of my own unhappiness. In hindsight, I was very depressed.

I remember one night so well. Flat on my back on my bedroom floor, I stared blankly at the ceiling fan. The anger twisted inside me. I could feel it thrashing—it was so painful—but I didn't know how to let it out. Tears slipping down my face, I dug my fingernails into my arm, pinching hard until little droplets of blood pooled under my fingernails.

Immediately, the pressure in my heart diminished. I could breathe! I had discovered a sweet relief, and I relied on this desperate measure a dozen

> *When I was thirteen years old, anger burned inside me.*

times in the following months. It was the only way I knew how to cope with school, my friends, my changing body . . . *my life*. Each time I did it, I grew more fearful of my own reckless behavior. I hid it from other people. I knew it wasn't healthy.

I came to my senses. With the help of my family and a therapist, I dug myself out of my emotional hole. I taught myself to see the goodness in my life and to let go of the things I could not control, and I found healthier outlets for my emotions. The experience showed me how to cope with life instead of running from it. Satisfied that I was "fixed," I moved forward.

I set up quite a successful life. In college, I felt like I had it all—a well-paying job, wonderful friends, true love, and an amazing education. But I was a terrible Fat Talker. I berated myself every single day for not being perfect. I would pull at my waistband and declare myself "fat." I felt guilty and angry when I skipped a workout. For eight torturous months, I logged the calorie content of every morsel of food that passed through my lips in a detailed spreadsheet on my computer. In my quest for perfection, I was making myself as miserable as I had been as a teenager.

My best friend Lauren is a wonderfully intelligent woman who I respect very much. One day, she sat me down and told me the blunt truth—I needed to either shape up or shut up. My Fat Talking was absolutely useless, Lauren told me. My lack of confidence kept me quiet in class, caused me to fight with my boyfriend, and generally held me back from experiencing life. My outlook was ruining my potential, my health, and my relationships. Lauren's straightforward approach snapped me out of my Fat Talk coma, and I vowed to stop Fat Talking. I quit the dirty habit cold turkey.

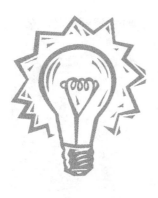

Instead of telling myself I was unhealthy and lazy, I told myself I was strong and beautiful. I repeated my positive mantras over and over again until I started to believe the messages. After ripping the batteries out of my scale, I stashed it under the bathroom sink. I quit calorie counting and began to eat intuitively. At the grocery store, I filled my cart with wholesome, natural foods instead of gimmicky diet foods.

I realized that my Fat Talk was a reflection of something much deeper than how I looked in the mirror. After years of beating myself up, I couldn't believe that the answer to a happier, healthier life was so simple. All I needed to do was treat myself with kindness, love, and patience. For the first time in a long time, I felt truly comfortable in my own skin.

Several years later, I was fighting a new kind of negative self-talk. At night, I took classes at a community college, and during the day, I had a demanding full-time job. The balancing act left me unhappy and anxious. Like clockwork, I experienced severe stomach pains every Sunday night. My husband worried that I was going to have a breakdown.

On a particularly stressful day, I was in a public restroom, and as I stared blankly into the mirror, I felt the urge to do something positive. I spontaneously scribbled "You are beautiful!" on a scrap piece of notebook paper and stuck it on the mirror. When I looked at the note, I felt lighter. I wondered who would find my note. Would it make her happy? Would it be the bright spot in her day? Would it feel like a message from the universe? I was giddy with excitement as I considered the possibilities of my note. I never dreamed that one little note was the start of something big.

That night, I posted a photograph of the note on my blog. Calling the mission Operation Beautiful, I urged other women in cyberspace to spread the love. My e-mail was immediately flooded with pictures and stories from women who posted their own notes on mirrors, magazines, and gym scales.

From my apartment in Orlando, Florida, I read e-mails from women in New York and California. Then, I started to hear from women in Canada, South America, Europe, and Asia. I received photographs of notes written in Chinese, German, and Spanish. A female soldier in Iraq sent me a note she posted in her barracks.

Everyone loved Operation Beautiful, and it was easy to see why. The Operation Beautiful do-gooders reported that posting the notes improved their mood. Some even said it changed their entire perspective on life. After all, the messages they wrote on the notes ("You are beautiful!" or "You deserve every kind of happiness!") were really messages to themselves.

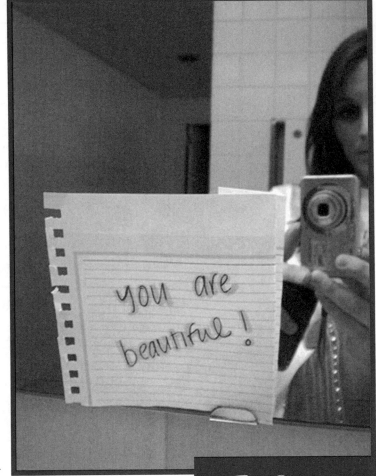

The Operation Beautiful note that started it all.

And then I started to hear from women who had *found* the notes. I read e-mails from women going through terrible divorces, teenagers feeling lost in high school, mothers coming to grips with their post-baby bodies, and girls in treatment clinics for eating disorders. For each woman, it seemed like the Operation Beautiful note was divine intervention. Women found an Operation Beautiful note when they needed it the most, and I started to believe that there are no coincidences. I realized that this story is about much more than a note left on a bathroom mirror.

My own personal experiences, as well as my involvement with Operation Beautiful, have convinced me that this life is nothing more than a series of lessons. Life is a learning experience, and we are all students. I truly believe that this random act of kindness is the springboard for discovering who you really are, what you really want, and how much you are capable of achieving.

Women are so attracted to Operation Beautiful for one reason: It works. Operation Beautiful is a positive, uplifting act that stamps out negative self-talk and encourages you to be the best version of yourself. The mission has nothing to do with how you look. It has nothing to do with your weight. Operation Beautiful is about who you are intrinsically as a person. It is about celebrating your unique personality, loving yourself *fully*, and letting go of any negativity that weighs you down. Whether you are the person posting the message or finding the note, Operation Beautiful transforms the way you see yourself.

Operation Beautiful is about one simple truth: You are beautiful . . . just the way you are!

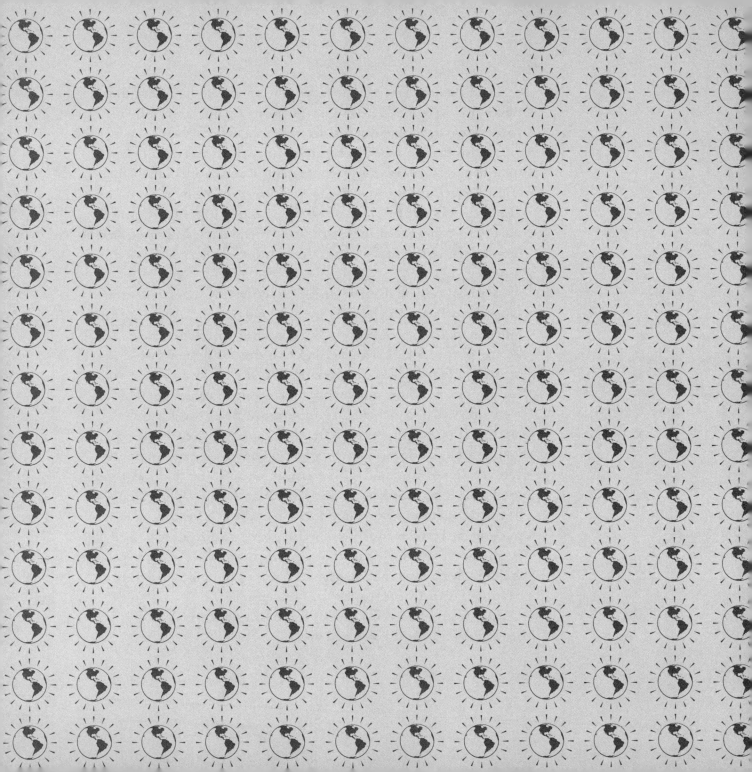

"I have posted this poem on various retail beauty counters around town over the past few months. I am traveling across the United States and South Pacific, and I intend to continue posting this note in my wake. I hope that whoever reads it will stop for just a moment and reflect on the message."

You are Beautiful
Just the Way You Are
Short or Skinny
Big or Tall
With Freckles, Acne,
Wrinkles & All
Young or Old
Black or White

& Even when your pants
get too tight
You are Beautiful
Just the Way You Are
Love Yourself &
all your flaws
Tell someone today
that they are Beautiful!

Lori S. • 52 • Calgary, Alberta, Canada

9

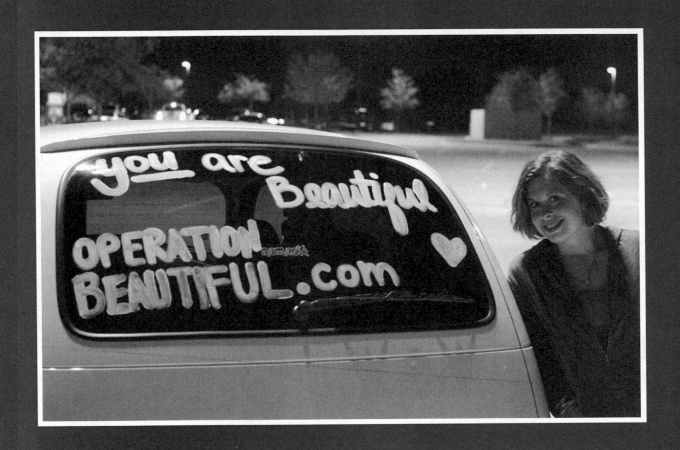

Kelsey Toney • 26 • Denton, Texas

"I had been trying to think of a way I could spread the Operation Beautiful mission farther . . . and faster! I got the idea to turn my car into an Operation Beautiful mobile. After writing the message in window chalk, I drove my car to the grocery store. I could not have been in the store for more than ten minutes, but when I came out, I found a scrap of grocery store receipt tucked under my wipers. It said, 'You made me smile. Thank you!' It's amazing how just a few short words can impact a person."

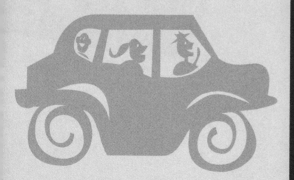

"I joined a new gym yesterday because I recently moved. Every gym I've ever joined requires that new members fill out a form related to their reasons for joining a gym and their corresponding fitness goals. In filling out the form, I checked the usual boxes that I wanted to work out to be healthy, relieve stress, improve athletic performance, etc. However, for the first time ever, I did not check the box that corresponded to the goal of losing weight. In the section about what I wanted to improve about my body, I drew a big 'X' over the section. I did this with a smile on my face, not because my body is perfect, but because I've recently come to accept my body the way it is and have realized that I don't need to be constantly fixated on ways I can improve it. In short, Operation Beautiful has reminded me to appreciate my body for what it can do and to embrace a healthy lifestyle with the goal of fitness in mind, rather than stressing over looks."

Shelley Ð. • 29 • Washington, Ð.C.

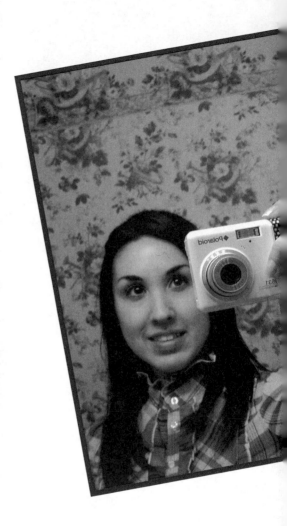

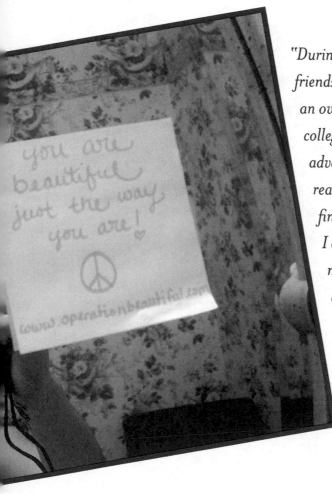

"During high school, I made excellent grades, had a lot of friends, and was even a dance team officer. I had always been an overachiever and a perfectionist from a young age. In college, these traits turned against me and worked to my disadvantage. I didn't know how to deal with the stresses of the real world, manage my hours between work and school, and find time to do homework when all I wanted to do was rest. I developed an eating disorder. Once I finally admitted to myself that I did have a problem, I began making positive changes in my life and was on the road to recovery.

Now there is no more counting every tedious calorie; it is a ridiculous waste of time. I would rather spend that time teaching my little sister how to bake. There is no more over-exercising for hours at the gym; I banished that gym membership. Instead, I take a walk with my mom and catch up on life. I am happy and eating disorder—free and could not wish for anything more.

I learned that there is so much more to life than counting calories and losing weight. If we could focus all this wasted energy into helping others who struggle with eating disorders, then we could change the way society views beauty and health. Being skinny doesn't define beauty; a natural and healthy person is beautiful."

Alicia Olivarez • 23 • San Antonio, Texas

"My hope is that someone stumbles across a real-life message in a bottle— a beautiful message—and it brightens their day."

Kath Younger • 27 •
Charlotte, North Carolina

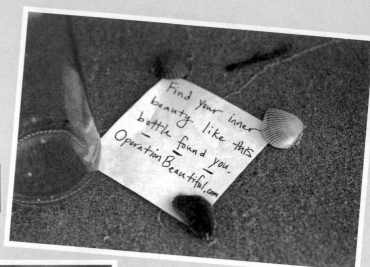

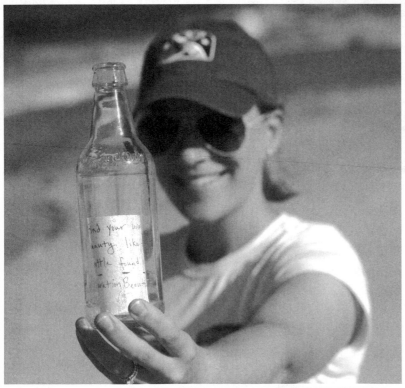

"One day, I was in a mall washroom, and although it was rather crowded, I wanted to leave an Operation Beautiful note. I quickly stuck it on the mirror and walked out. Then, this girl, who had been curiously looking on in the washroom, taps me on the shoulder in tears and gives me this huge hug, thanking me. It made me tear up as well. It was an incredible feeling!"

Brooke Vickery • 16 • Richmond Hill, Ontario, Canada

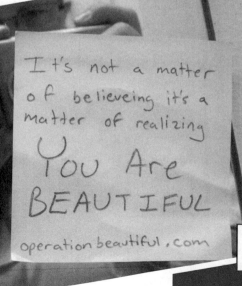

It's not a matter of believeing it's a matter of realizing YOU ARE BEAUTIFUL

operation beautiful.com

"It took me a while to think of something that I believe in to write on this note. Just thinking about this helped me so much. I realized that I really am beautiful, and so is everyone else, because no one is alike. It's the things that make us different that make us beautiful."

Lisa Klatkiewicz • 21 • Seymour, Wisconsin

15

"I was visiting a bookstore to pick up some books about dieting and fitness. I was very upset with the sort of things these books were suggesting—I can't live on vegetables and spend two hours at the gym every day. Then, I opened another book and found a note that read: 'You are beautiful no matter what the scale says. Google Operation Beautiful.' It was . . . surprising and very pleasant. I felt myself warm inside, just like I feel every time when I'm writing stories or poems—the strange feeling that I am not alone, and someone cared to leave this note so I could find it."

Alia Luna Miroshnichenko • 19 •
Guelph, Ontario, Canada

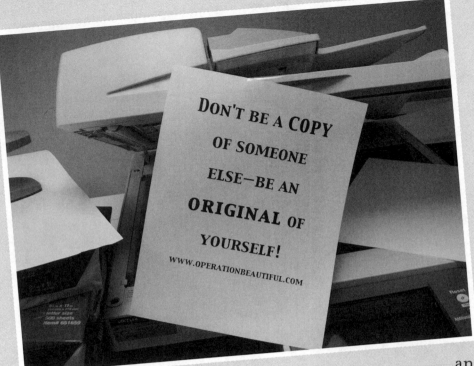

DON'T BE A COPY OF SOMEONE ELSE—BE AN **ORIGINAL** OF YOURSELF!

WWW.OPERATIONBEAUTIFUL.COM

Mary S. • 33 • Minneapolis, Minnesota

"I just found an Operation Beautiful note last night on the bathroom stall at Wal-Mart. I was trying on clothes and noticed that I'd gained a lot of weight over the last year. I was being so incredibly negative and hard on myself that I didn't feel like anything could make me feel better. But then I saw the Post-it, and it honestly made my day. It made me totally reevaluate my way of thinking. Now I'm back on track, working on getting in shape, and continuing to spread the Operation Beautiful message to keep myself positive. This way, I can reach my goals while helping others!"

Carrie Finn • 22 • Ottawa, Ontario, Canada

17

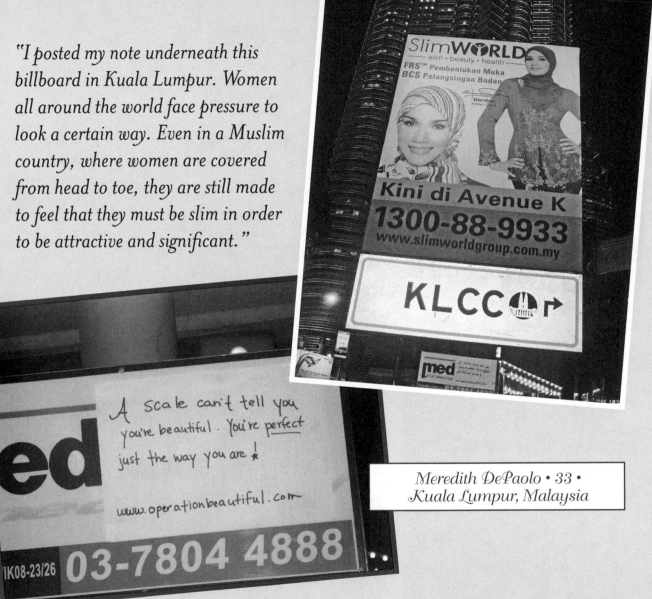

"*I posted my note underneath this billboard in Kuala Lumpur. Women all around the world face pressure to look a certain way. Even in a Muslim country, where women are covered from head to toe, they are still made to feel that they must be slim in order to be attractive and significant.*"

Meredith DePaolo • 33 •
Kuala Lumpur, Malaysia

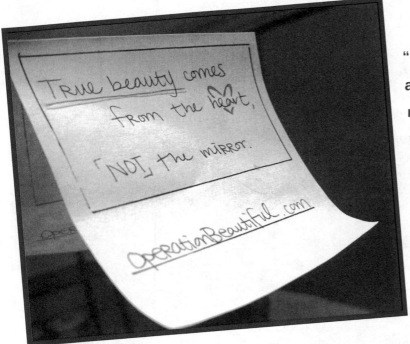

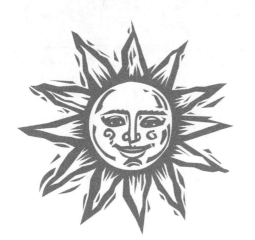

"Operation Beautiful has created a whole new view on the world for me. Recently, I actually found a wonderful note in a book at the library. It said, 'Everyone is beautiful in unique ways. View with positivity and the world will look different. View with positivity and more happiness will come your way. Remember, you're beautiful inside and out. It's the attitude and perspective that changes everything.' After reading this note, I realized that I really should not spend my time—my life—worrying about appearance. It's about my happiness and the happiness of people that I love. After finding this inspiring note, I started to leave notes myself. I've been leaving them in public places like bathrooms, locker rooms, and grocery shops."

Junghwa • 20 • Los Angeles, California

"*We bought permanent markers and an array of Post-it notes. Sneaking into the bathroom after school, we decorated the mirror with Post-it notes with sayings such as 'You are beautiful,' 'Smile,' 'Dream.' The end of the year is fast approaching so we were determined to make it a good one!*"

Britt and Lily • 16 • Australia

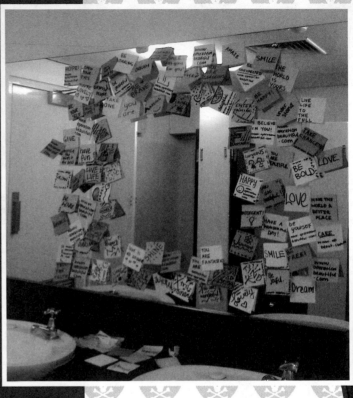

"Exactly twelve months had passed since I had left inpatient treatment [for an eating disorder]. And, as God would have it, I had just reached my ideal body weight. I was really struggling with accepting this 'new' body and was hating everything about how I looked and felt. I scrolled through the

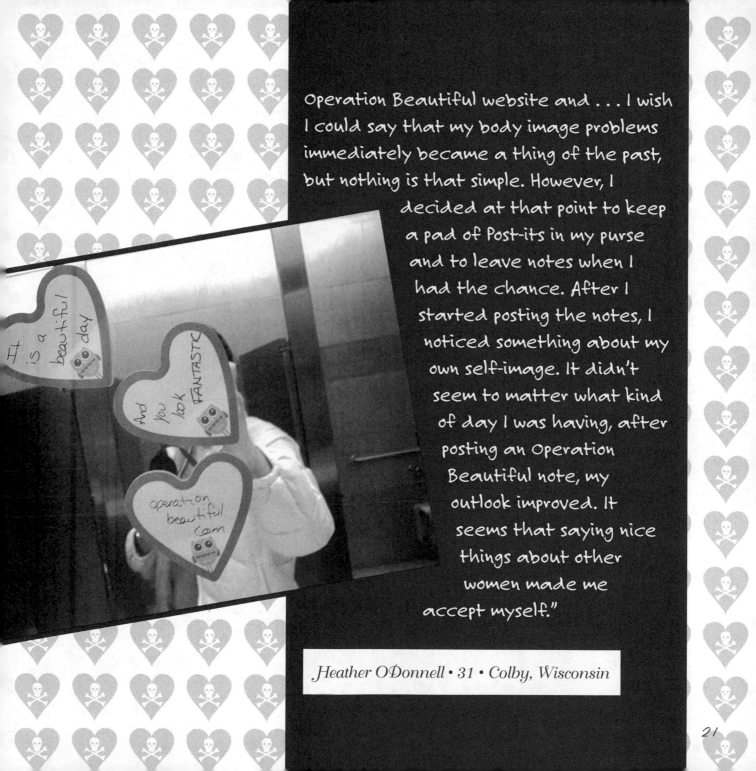

Operation Beautiful website and . . . I wish I could say that my body image problems immediately became a thing of the past, but nothing is that simple. However, I decided at that point to keep a pad of Post-its in my purse and to leave notes when I had the chance. After I started posting the notes, I noticed something about my own self-image. It didn't seem to matter what kind of day I was having, after posting an Operation Beautiful note, my outlook improved. It seems that saying nice things about other women made me accept myself."

Heather O'Donnell • 31 • Colby, Wisconsin

"I am seventeen years old, live in Canada, and was diagnosed with bulimia when I was fourteen. I began my first diet when I was eight. I have spent my entire life working to be 'perfect' and thin. It has ruined my life. My teeth have almost no enamel left on them, my heart rate and blood pressure goes from too high to too low weekly. I get ECGs and blood tests at least once a month. I have spent my last two summers in hospitals and have missed part of grades ten, eleven, and twelve due to being hospitalized. I can't stand up for very long without my vision going black and getting dizzy. My hair fell out a few years back. My fingernails turn blue and I'm always cold. I can't go out with my friends anymore; I get too tired. I have wasted so much time and truly put my health at risk, and I still can't stop.

The reason I'm writing is because on Friday, I was at my weekly hospital checkup and one of my therapists made me eat a five-hundred-calorie meal, which I haven't done in ages, to 'densensitize' me. I was on my way to the bathroom to throw it up after my appointment. I had just locked the stall when I saw a sticky note on the back of the door. It said, 'You're beautiful. You're good enough.' No one has ever said that to me. I didn't throw up that day. It was the first time I ate something solid and did not throw it up in years."

Vit • 17 • Toronto, Ontario, Canada

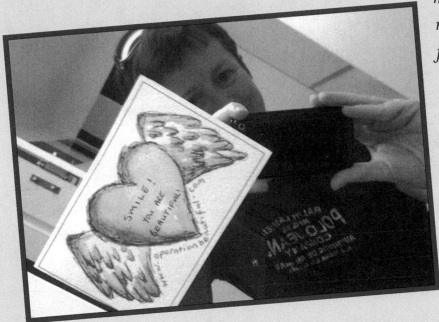

"*The day I sat down with a pen in my hand to write my first note I felt a shiver of excitement. I felt a little bit self-conscious, worried that if I was caught I would be thought of as 'odd,' but I did it anyway. I was hoping that someone somewhere reading one of my notes would feel this random message had come at just the point that they needed it. What I didn't expect was the feeling I would get from participating. I walked around with a spring in my step and butterflies in my tummy like a kid on Christmas Eve. Being part of Operation Beautiful has been such a fun experience. If even one person feels good about themselves after finding one of my notes, then it is a success in my eyes.*"

Gina Haynham • 36 • Australia

"I worked in my local gym as a cleaner. I was doing 'locker checks,' where we check the lockers for rubbish and lost property, when I found a yellow note. Written on it in blue marker was 'Smile! You are beautiful.' I felt ten times happier! I had been feeling down because I am surrounded by mirrors and gym bunnies as I work, and the note made my day a whole lot better. Thank you to whoever left me that note. It also gave me the courage to quit my job the following day!"

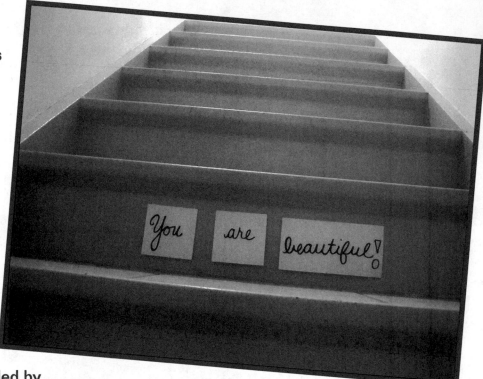

Karina Diaz • 22 • Manhattan, New York

Alice G. • 20 • Halifax, England

Michelle • 34 • Hong Kong

"One day, I was in the elevator at work and decided to post an Operation Beautiful note on the buttons, hoping someone who needed it would find it. Imagine my surprise when I arrived at work the next day and spotted my note inside the security guard's station. He loved my note and kept it! I was aiming for a woman, but I guess a man needed my message, too!"

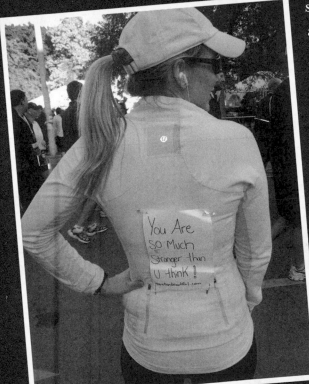

"I posted this Operation Beautiful note on my back while running a half marathon in Toronto. To my surprise, I had about fifteen people come up to me during the half marathon, high-five me, and tell me how amazing my sign was. I was even more amazed by how much it lifted my spirits when I felt like giving up."

Angela Liddon • 26 • Toronto, Ontario, Canada

"Thanks to Operation Beautiful, my life was saved. I used to be very self-conscious about my body. I had been put down and made fun of for not being skinny and fit like the rest of the girls. I was so fed up with it, I started contemplating suicide. On one of my better days, I went to class and on my chair was a note. I was worried it was something hateful. Instead I opened it to see a note that read, 'Take a rest, you deserve it. Remember, you are beautiful in every way!' I found more random notes scrawled on chalkboards, taped to a desk, and even on lockers. I started to feel so much better. After that, I tore up my suicide notes. I'm trying to be an inspiration to younger kids who might be struggling like I did. My library gives out free bookmarks geared toward younger kids, and I took a few of the bookmarks and wrote 'You are beautiful!' on the backs. I felt amazing."

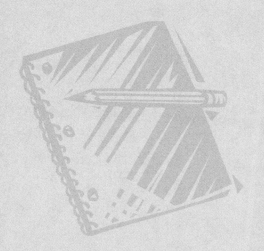

Sarah • 18 • Illinois

Chapter 2

Fat Talk

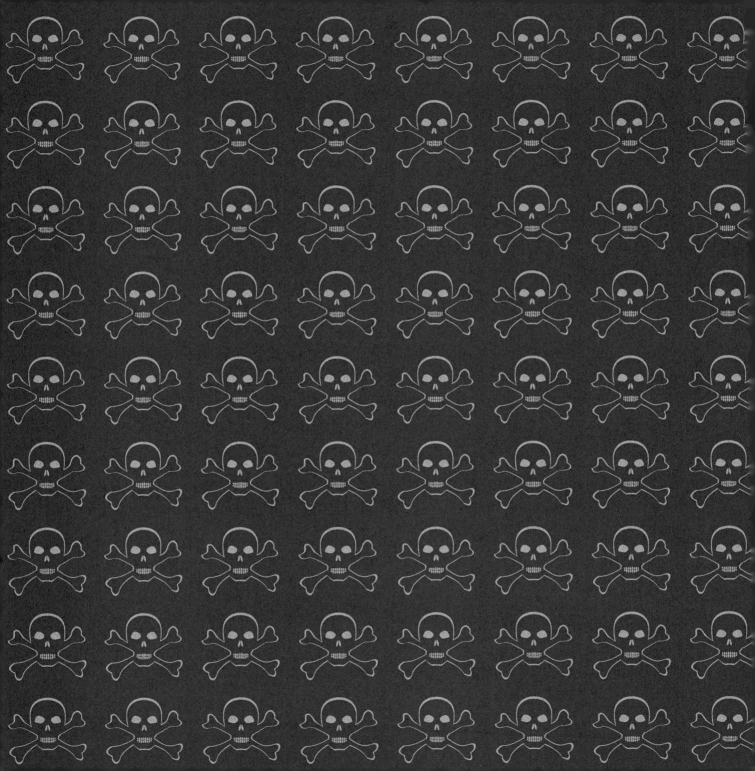

The Fat Talk Trap

*W*hen Brandi Evans was a teenager, she easily maintained a healthy weight. "But in college, everything changed," Brandi says. "I wasn't taking care of myself, eating the right foods, or working out." She gained thirty pounds by her sophomore year.

"I broke down in a dressing room while shopping with my mom during Christmas vacation," Brandi remembers. "I was so unhappy with how I felt, how I looked, and how I was treating myself." As Brandi struggled to improve her eating and exercise habits, she fell into the Fat Talk trap. "I became very critical of myself." She showered herself with negative messages, put pressure on herself to be perfect, and felt guilty when she fell off the "diet bandwagon."

After joining Weight Watchers, Brandi lost—and kept off—most of the weight she had gained. The Fat Talk, however, wouldn't go away. "That number on the scale had so much power over me for

> *That number on the scale had so much power over me.*

the past few years. The lower it was, the better my day," says Brandi. "If it was up, and I didn't know why, it could put me in a terrible mood."

Over time, Brandi shifted her focus away from counting calories, points, and pounds, prioritizing her overall health and happiness. "My thinking had to change in order to maintain my weight loss in a healthy way," she admits. Brandi also began to post Operation Beautiful notes encouraging other women to stop Fat Talking. "Those messages allowed me to stop critiquing myself and focus on the things I could do," Brandi says.

When she eliminated Fat Talk from her vocabulary, she was amazed at the positive effect it had on her outlook. "Operation Beautiful has the power to really change people from the inside out, and that's the way to make lasting lifestyle changes," Brandi says. "It's not about losing weight, gaining muscle, or fitting in my old jeans from high school. I'm taking better care of myself because I deserve it."

Brandi Evans • 26 • Pembroke, Virginia

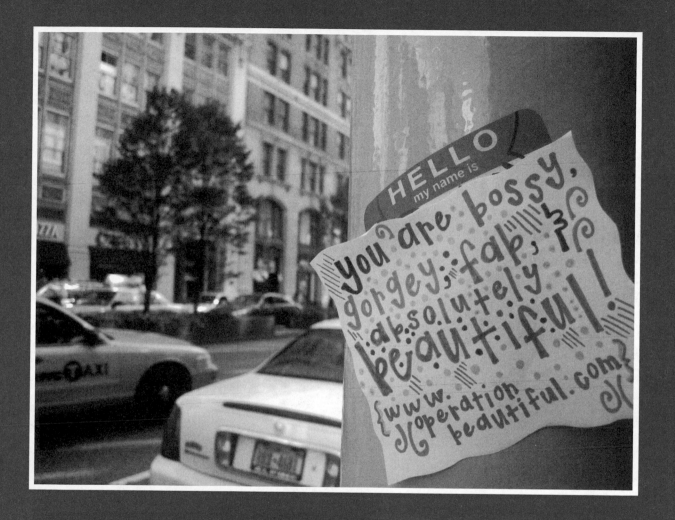

Brooke McCallion • 18 •
New York , New York

"I posted this note on the fountain in front of the Pantheon, one of my very favorite places in Rome. It seemed fitting to put it on such an ancient building with such a rich history. I stepped back and watched several tourists see the note and read it. It made me feel good to know that the note had the ability to reach so many different people from all walks of life, speaking all languages. If it made a difference to only one person, it is enough."

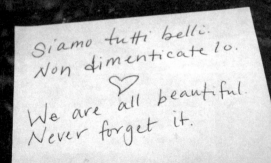

Siamo tutti belli.
Non dimenticate lo.
♡
We are all beautiful.
Never forget it.

Ellen • 20 • Rome, Italy

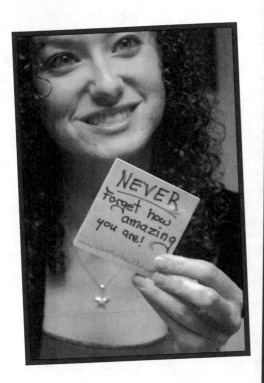

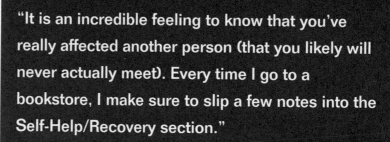

"It is an incredible feeling to know that you've really affected another person (that you likely will never actually meet). Every time I go to a bookstore, I make sure to slip a few notes into the Self-Help/Recovery section."

Amy Brooks • 22 • Ringwood, New Jersey

"I was at Borders looking for a self-help book that my therapist (who I had just started seeing) recommended. Imagine my surprise when I found a Post-it stuck to the inside cover of the book *Binge No More* that said, 'NEVER forget how amazing you are!' I was so overwhelmed with emotion that I started to cry on the spot. That little note made me realize just how much I've taken myself for granted over the years. Whoever wrote that note . . . thank you! Thank you for helping this broken girl start to heal. I have been binge-free for three months now."

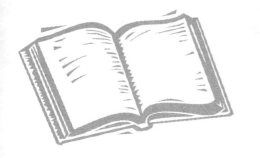

Christina • 21 • New Jersey

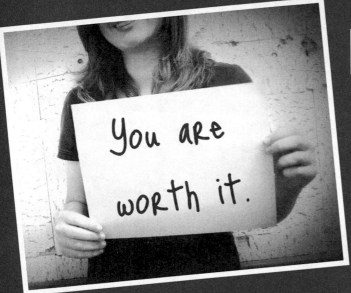

Amelia C. • 21 • Sandy Hook, Kentucky

"I know it's easy to feel worthless, and sometimes it helps just to be reminded of the truth."

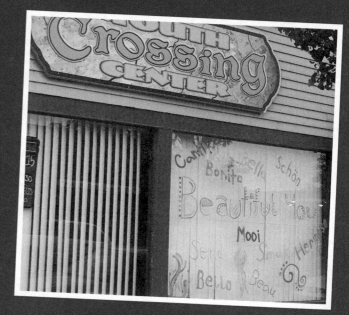

"This youth center is on the main street of our little town of Springville. The idea was to create a safe place for kids to hang out with friends after school and build relationships with adults who care about them. A group of about ten students came up with the idea to decorate the window to let their friends know that they are beautiful on the inside, where it counts."

Becca E. • 36 • Springville, New York

"For seven years, I struggled with my body image. I was the biggest 'Fat Talker.' But then I stumbled upon Operation Beautiful, and the Fat Talk ended. People around me actually noticed that I was happier and more confident. This has helped me see that I am beautiful and I was beautiful, even at my highest weight of 220 pounds. I was beautiful as a size eighteen, and I'm beautiful now as a size six. Beauty is not what you see on the outside. . . ."

Kathryn D. • 23 • Chestertown, Maryland

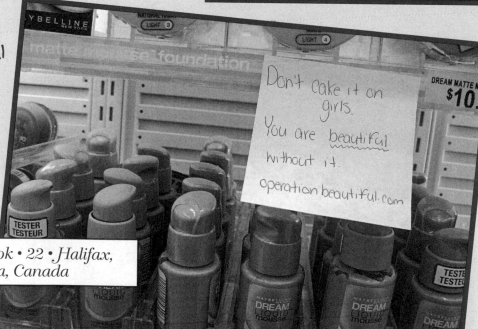

insatiable
a young mother's struggle with anorexia

"It only takes ONE person to change Your life... You" - Ruth Casey

You aRE Beautiful, amazing & strong!

www.operationbeautiful.com

Don't cake it on girls.
You are beautiful without it.
operation beautiful.com

Christine Newhook • 22 • Halifax, Nova Scotia, Canada

"I am fifty-eight years old, and I never use the 'F' (fat) word, but there is the aging thing. No matter how hard we try to hide it, by the time we reach a certain age it's there, especially when you're standing in the ladies' room under those awful fluorescent lights. There I was, at a mall in North Sydney, Nova Scotia, yesterday, digging in my purse for my lipstick. I look up and there on the mirror I see the first of three Post-its I was to spot that day in the mall. It said, 'Smile—you're beautiful!' I stood in front of it for a while—and yes, I was smiling—and wondering why such a small gesture could make me feel so good! This person didn't know me, didn't see me—it wasn't even meant for me, personally. But it really made my day. I have since picked up a Post-it pad and am spreading my own sunshine. And that makes me smile, too!"

Donna T. • 58 • Sydney, Nova Scotia, Canada

Justine Moavero • 27 • Orlando, Florida

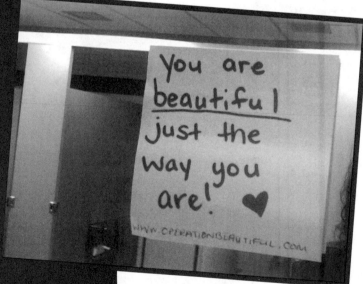

You are beautiful just the way you are! ♥
WWW.OPERATIONBEAUTIFUL.COM

36

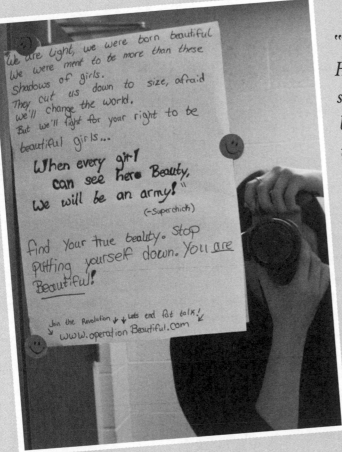

"This was taken at Forest View Psychiatric Hospital. I was there for an eating disorder support group. I was really stressing out before the meeting. I had a hard couple of weeks, and all I wanted to do was run back into my eating disorder. Before the meeting started, I went to the bathroom to take a deep breath and calm down. As I was in there, I thought of the pens and paper in my bag and quickly made up this note for the mirror. I don't know if anyone else was affected by it, but it meant a lot to me. I told myself in the note what I most needed to hear. I was able to remind myself that I was going to be all right, that even if I didn't feel it right then, I am beautiful and loved. And I didn't need to stand in the bathroom and beat myself up like I normally would have before the meetings.

My hope in posting the note on the mirror was that the next struggling girl in the bathroom would see the note and be reminded that she was loved and beautiful, too."

Bethany M. • 20 • Grand Rapids, Michigan

37

The Real Deal with Fat Talk

Fat Talk isn't about being overweight.
In fact, Fat Talk has nothing to do
with your size at all.

- Women engage in Fat Talk for a variety of reasons, as it allows them to "express emotions, seek social reassurance, create an in-group with friends, excuse certain eating behaviors, and manage impressions," according to Dr. Denise Martz, a clinical psychologist who has spent more than twenty years studying body image, eating disorders, and Fat Talk.

- Fat Talk is habitual, meaning that women often don't realize they are doing it. Fat Talk has become a knee-jerk reaction to eating an indulgent meal, trying on bathing suits, or even getting dressed in the morning.

- Fat Talk triggers unhealthy behaviors, whether the comments are consciously processed or not. Putting yourself down verbally creates reverse inertia in all aspects of your life. Instead of inspiring you to get healthier, Fat Talk will motivate you to overeat, skip your workouts, and stay involved in toxic relationships. Additionally, even if you don't "hear" your own Fat Talk, your friends

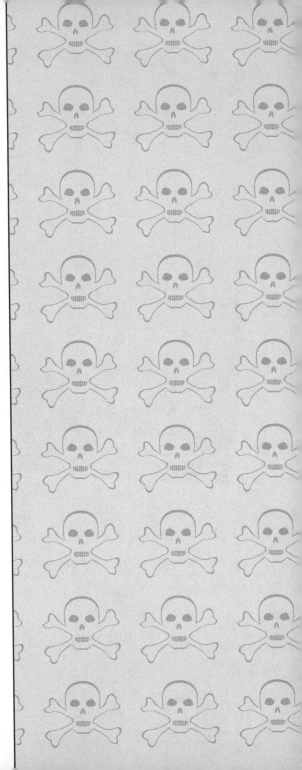

and family members will, and it harms them emotionally, spiritually, and physically as well.

- Women use Fat Talk to bond socially. Women Fat Talk with their friends, and mothers Fat Talk with their daughters. Fat Talk is contagious, and if one woman does it, the next may feel compelled to engage in the behavior, too. "Fat Talk has become a form of chitchat," says Dr. Susan Albers, a psychologist who specializes in relationship and weight issues. Dr. Albers has observed that women will often mirror a friend's Fat Talk. "We tend to follow other people's leads, particularly those who are close to us."

- Fat Talk is also a coping mechanism. Our society places pressure on us to look a certain way, and when we don't, we often react by shaming ourselves with Fat Talk. The behavior is an unhealthy and unproductive form of venting. Through Fat Talk, we can express our fears or insecurities, and other people usually accept this Fat Talk and respond with praise, which reinforces the behavior (for example, one girl says, "That model is so skinny; look how fat I am in comparison!" and the other girl responds, "You aren't fat; you are so tiny!").

- Fat Talk allows us to hide our true emotions. Instead of admitting we feel sad, guilty, or lonely, women often pick apart their physical features.

"When you say, 'I feel fat,' many people will nod sympathetically," says Dr. Albers, who authored the book *50 Ways to Soothe Yourself Without Food*. "In this context, it is used as a shorthand way of communicating how you feel. It's interesting that we pin insecure and uncomfortable feelings onto our bodies instead of identifying the real reasons underlying the discomfort."

- Fat Talk is an expected behavior. "Imagine walking into a room and stating that you are happy or comfortable with your body. How would people look at you?" says Dr. Albers. "Unfortunately, it is a cultural norm to be dissatisfied with your body."

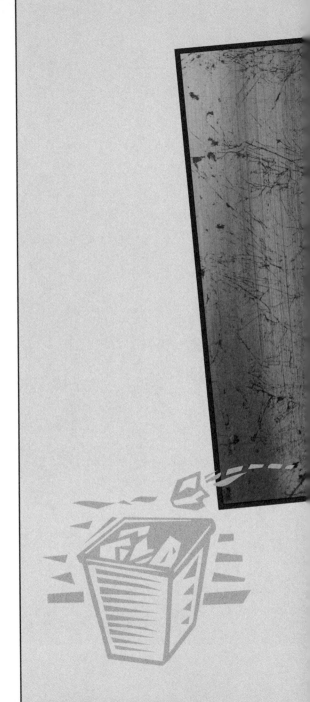

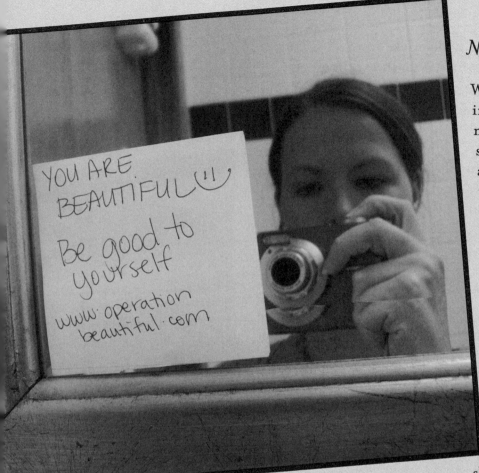

YOU ARE
BEAUTIFUL☺
Be good to
yourself
www·operation
beautiful·com

Sarah F. • 27 • Louisville, Kentucky

No More Negativity

When Sarah set out to improve her health, she lost more than seventy pounds— she also dropped her negative attitude. "From the time I was a child, I had always been negative about my self-image," she says. "It's not surprising that I became an incredibly unhealthy adult. The mind is so powerful, and if you let negative thoughts fill your head, they will devour you."

Sarah's journey began on the eve of her twenty-fifth birthday. She was depressed and out of shape. "All I did was go to work, come home, and lay on the couch," she remembers. "When I did go out with friends, I was uncomfortable in my own skin. I felt like the 'fat friend' in my group, and when I opened my wedding album, I cried. I even called myself the 'fat bride' as I looked at the pictures." Tired of her negative self-talk, Sarah decided she needed to overhaul her life.

"Something in my head finally clicked, and I decided that enough was enough," Sarah recalls. "I wanted to enjoy the rest of my life. It was finally about more than weight loss."

Instead of relying on vending machines and fast food restaurants for her meals, Sarah began to eat breakfast at home, pack her lunch, and exercise. Almost immediately, the little changes started to add up. "Not only was I losing weight, but I felt so much healthier," she says. "I never focused on reaching a 'goal weight.' When we focus too much on numbers, it defeats the purpose of getting healthy. What matters is that you find a place where you are comfortable with your body and are happy."

To improve her mental health, Sarah made lists of all the wonderful things in her life. She also jotted down the benefits of reducing her cholesterol and blood pressure. "To this day, I talk to myself in the mirror!" she says. "When I accomplish something, I reinforce it by reminding myself how great I'm doing. If something troublesome comes, I tell my reflection that everything will be fine."

The most important change for Sarah was when she stopped believing there was "a finish line." Instead, Sarah knows that "staying healthy and happy is a process that never ends. We have to keep challenging ourselves to stay focused and positive."

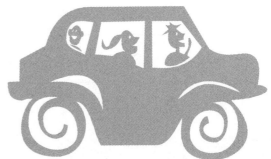

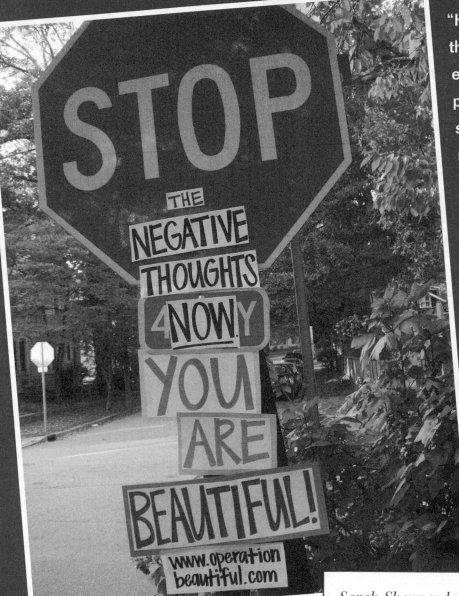

STOP THE NEGATIVE THOUGHTS 4 NOW. YOU ARE BEAUTIFUL!

www.operation beautiful.com

"Hundreds of cars pass through this four-way stop every day. If just one person takes a second to step back from their road rage and realize the beauty of life from the words I posted on this stop sign, I have succeeded. Operation Beautiful stands for everything I believe. The more that we can start to appreciate our bodies and stop comparing ourselves to others, the closer we can all come to living happier, more beautiful lives."

Sarah Sheppard • 19 • Richmond, Virginia

"For a long time, I felt like my body wasn't good enough, like I didn't have enough of a chest, and like I wasn't ever going to fit in. I've always been really skinny, and although most people don't seem to realize it, 'You're a waif! I mean, I always knew you were skinny, but you're just really waifish!' is not a compliment. I'm finally confident enough to accept that I am different, and I'm proud of that. I really don't care what people think about me, as long as I'm true to myself and my standards."

Jenn • 16 • Alexandria, Virginia

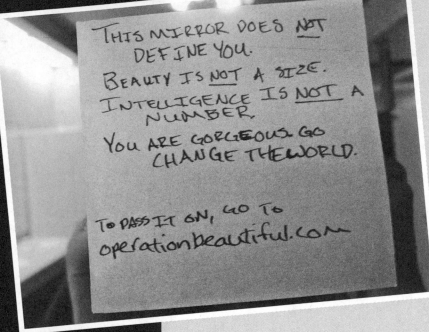

THIS MIRROR DOES NOT DEFINE YOU.
BEAUTY IS NOT A SIZE.
INTELLIGENCE IS NOT A NUMBER.
YOU ARE GORGEOUS. GO CHANGE THE WORLD.

TO PASS IT ON, GO TO operationbeautiful.com

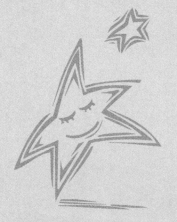

Crystal Newberry • 28 • Toronto, Ontario, Canada

You are Beautiful ...yes You!!!

"When I have a negative thought, I remember the Operation Beautiful notes I've posted. I get a rush of happiness every time!"

"I have lost eighty pounds, but I continue to struggle with my self-image every day. I recently decided to put away my scale for an entire month. I no longer want to have my day ruled by what number shows up on the scale. I am worth more."

Syl • 33 • Calgary, Alberta, Canada

Good Morning Beautiful You have accomplished so much. Stay Strong, be Proud! Operationbeautiful.com

"I left a note rolled up in my bus fare for the person who counts the money at the end of the day. I heard from someone I know at the bus company that the note kept people at the office happy for days! Operation Beautiful has changed my thinking on a daily basis. Before, I woke up dreading another dreary day. Now, I wake up and find the positive in every single thing that happens in my day! I have started helping older people on and off the bus each and every time, too. It makes me feel good that I can bring a smile to someone's face who might not have smiled otherwise. It makes me realize that I am special and more beautiful than I ever imagined I could be."

Kathy • 48 • Medina, Ohio

Polyrhythm • 18 • West Midlands, United Kingdom

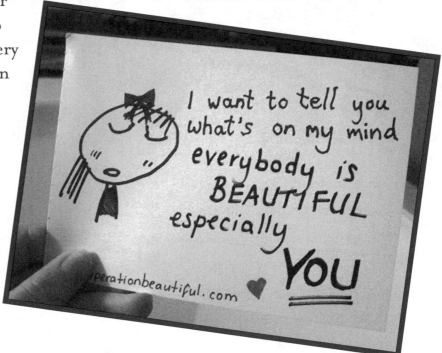

46

Jennifer Grigsby • 30 • Bono, Arkansas

"I took my eight-year-old son to swimming lessons. I had my pads of Post-its and marker, and I had already filled out a bunch with various inspirational messages. I told my son about Operation Beautiful and he got very excited and wanted to help me. We put up blue and green stickies everywhere we went that day: in bathrooms, inside magazines, and on a box of Slim-Fast. We had such a fun time doing it, and he wants to create more notes and go on another posting spree!"

Believe that
You CAN and
You will!

operationbeautiful.com

"I've done things I never thought I could do, and it's all because I stopped thinking, 'When I lose ten pounds . . .' I wish I had listened to everyone who told me I was okay the way I was. I am worth it. I want others who have self-doubt to feel as happy and beautiful as I do now. I want them to stop Fat Talk and learn self-love and acceptance."

B. A. Coyne • 22 • Vancouver, British Columbia, Canada

47

"Although I still personally have a really hard time believing the positive messages, I think Operation Beautiful is something that can contribute to changing the way we view our bodies. I slipped this note inside another girl's laundry bag. I know she has an eating disorder, and I hope this note made her day a little brighter and helped her see how beautiful she already is."

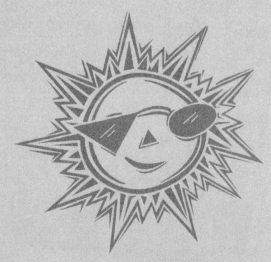

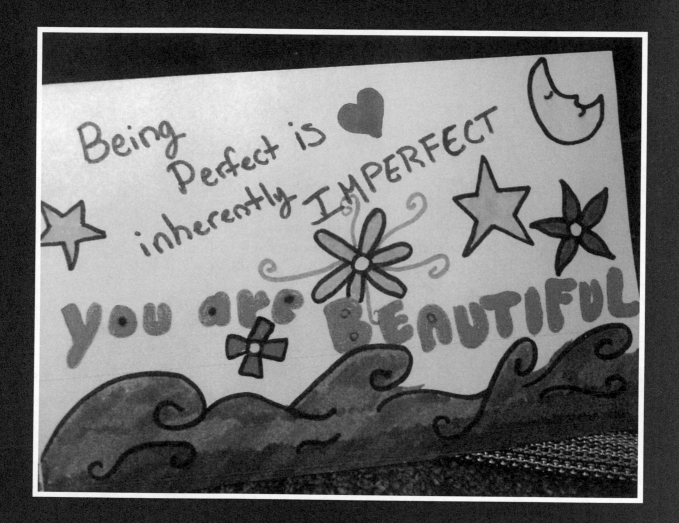

Being Perfect is inherently IMPERFECT

YOU are BEAUTIFUL

Pam S. • 18 • Connecticut

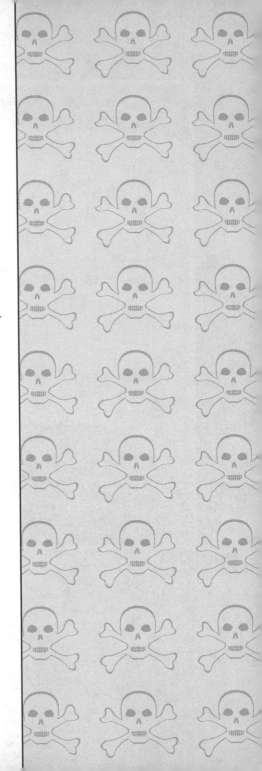

Fighting Fat Talk

Fat Talking is a bad habit that you can break. Here's how:

- Healthy living is the culmination of many positive choices. Instead of beating yourself up over one indulgent meal or a skipped workout, consider your lifestyle in terms of a week or month. If you've truly fallen off the healthy bandwagon and slipped back into unhealthy behaviors, carefully evaluate why this has occurred and what positive lessons you can learn from the experience. Remember that each meal and each day is a new beginning, so start implementing more positive choices right away! Also, negative self-talk only reinforces your unhealthy behavior, so cut yourself some slack and remind yourself that your journey is not about perfection but progress.

- Consciously correct yourself if you Fat Talk. "Replace negative self-talk with balanced, believable thoughts," advises Dr. Joy Jacobs, a body image expert who serves on the Professional Advisory Panel for Families Empowered and Supporting Treatment of Eating Disorders (F.E.A.S.T.).

- Stop your Fat Talk in its tracks! In addition to consciously correcting yourself, try wearing a rubber band around your wrist and give it a firm "*snap!*" whenever you feel a negative thought creeping in. Think of it like coating your nails in spicy polish when you're trying to stop biting them! The rubber band technique is a gentle physical reminder of the internal damage you are doing to yourself when you Fat Talk.

- Identify the real issue behind your Fat Talk. Is it really about your body or is it about something else entirely—like an emotion you're having trouble expressing? Many women use Fat Talk as a way to express sadness or frustration. Find a more positive outlet for your emotions, such as talking to a friend, writing in your diary, or exercising.

- Make a list of your positive qualities—both inside and out—and tape them to your bathroom mirror so you can read it whenever you need a boost. Do not be ashamed to celebrate your amazing qualities!

- Refrain from making judgments about yourself or other people based on appearance. Realize that complimentary statements about someone's looks ("You look great! Have you lost weight?") can be just as damaging as Fat Talk. Focus on personalities and achievements, not dress size.

- Help others to help yourself. Post an Operation Beautiful note, call a friend, or volunteer at a charity. "I wish that women would put more effort into taking care of themselves, taking care of each other, and trying to make the world a better place instead of Fat Talking," says Dr. Martz.

Redefine Beautiful

Little girls all over the world love to play with Barbie and dress her in pretty outfits. But if Barbie was alive, her waist would be smaller than a woman with severe anorexia nervosa. Barbie's body weight would be so low that she would be unable to menstruate.

As we grow older, the media continues to reinforce this Thin Ideal. We're bombarded with images of airbrushed celebrities and models with unrealistic, unattainable bodies. We spend billions on products that promise to slim our thighs, whiten our teeth, shine our hair, and smooth our skin. As women, we've been trained to believe that we're never good enough.

With such unrealistic ideals to emulate, it's unsurprising that 81 percent of ten-year-olds report that they are afraid of being fat. Half of teenage girls admit to extreme dieting behaviors such as fasting, purging, or sabotaging their food. Unbelievably, researchers have found that 50 percent of young adults would rather be hit by a truck than be fat.

Even pregnant women are expected to conform to the Thin Ideal. "When I was pregnant with my second child, people frequently commented that I looked huge," recalls Christina. "A perfect stranger told me that I needed to cut back on the snacks." Upon catching a glimpse of Christina's pregnant stomach, her mother-in-law remarked that her stretch marks

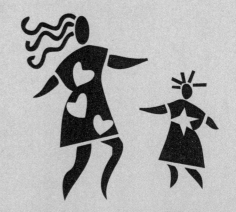

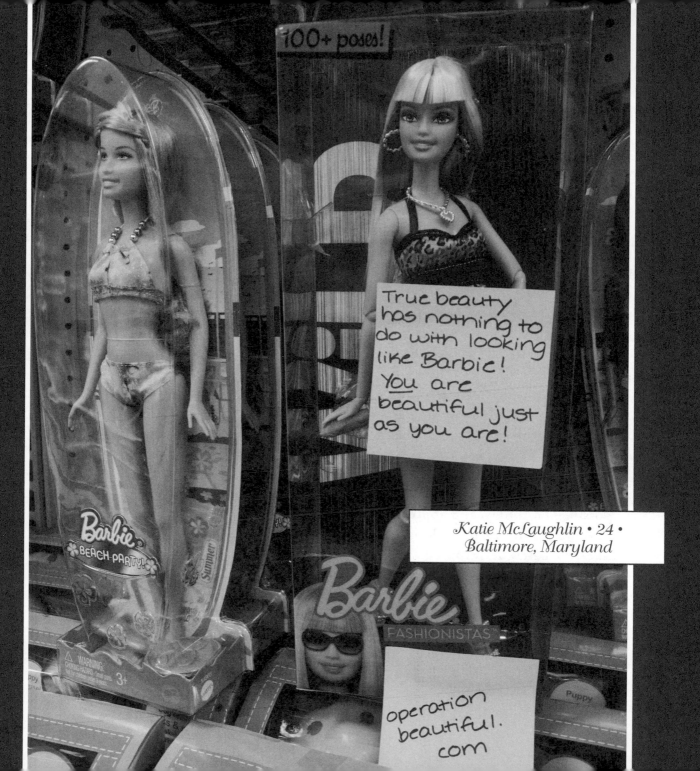

were "awful." "It tore at my self-esteem," says Christina. "I knew that my body would never be the same as it was before."

After the birth of my second child, I was having a difficult time coming to terms with my new body," Christina says. "There are a few more curves, twice the stretch marks, and a little more ripple on my tummy. I thought myself to be ugly. I don't know exactly when it changed, but one day I realized that this new body of mine has grown, given birth to, and nourished two beautiful children. The stretch marks on my body are a physical reminder of those short eighteen months that they grew inside and the time they spent as nurslings. I have come to realize how beautiful that is. My stretch marks only add to the beauty that is already there."

It's time for us to let go of this impossible Thin Ideal and appreciate our bodies for the amazing things they can do. We must create a new definition of beauty, a definition that encompasses more than our physical appearance and focuses on our inner light. This is a gift we can give ourselves and future generations of women.

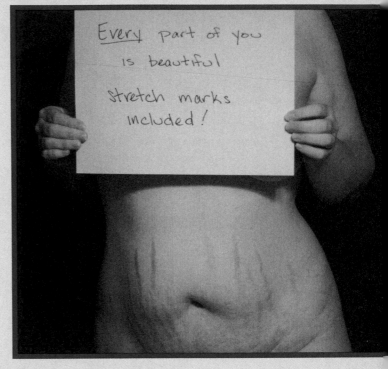

Christina A. • 28 • Austin, Texas

54

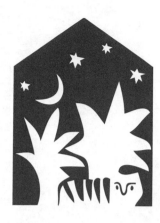

Sheila Viers • 28 • Santa Monica, California

"I have run the gamut of metabolism-related health problems. I've had thyroid problems, hormonal problems, digestion problems—but I've dealt with them all and realized that 99 percent of my issues were directly related to things I was doing to or putting into my body. These days, I would say that I have righted the self-esteem/body-image issues that I once had. I have reached a place where I am happy with all that I am, both inside and out. I had to get over a lot of stuff before I came to that good-feeling place. To be totally honest, I know that as I continue to grow personally, that mind-body relationship will still get better and better. I am a student of life, and each day provides new insight and opportunity to grow."

SELF CONFIDENCE IS THE ROCK SOLID FOUNDATION TO A SKYSCRAPER OF HAPPINESS.

—SHEILA VIERS

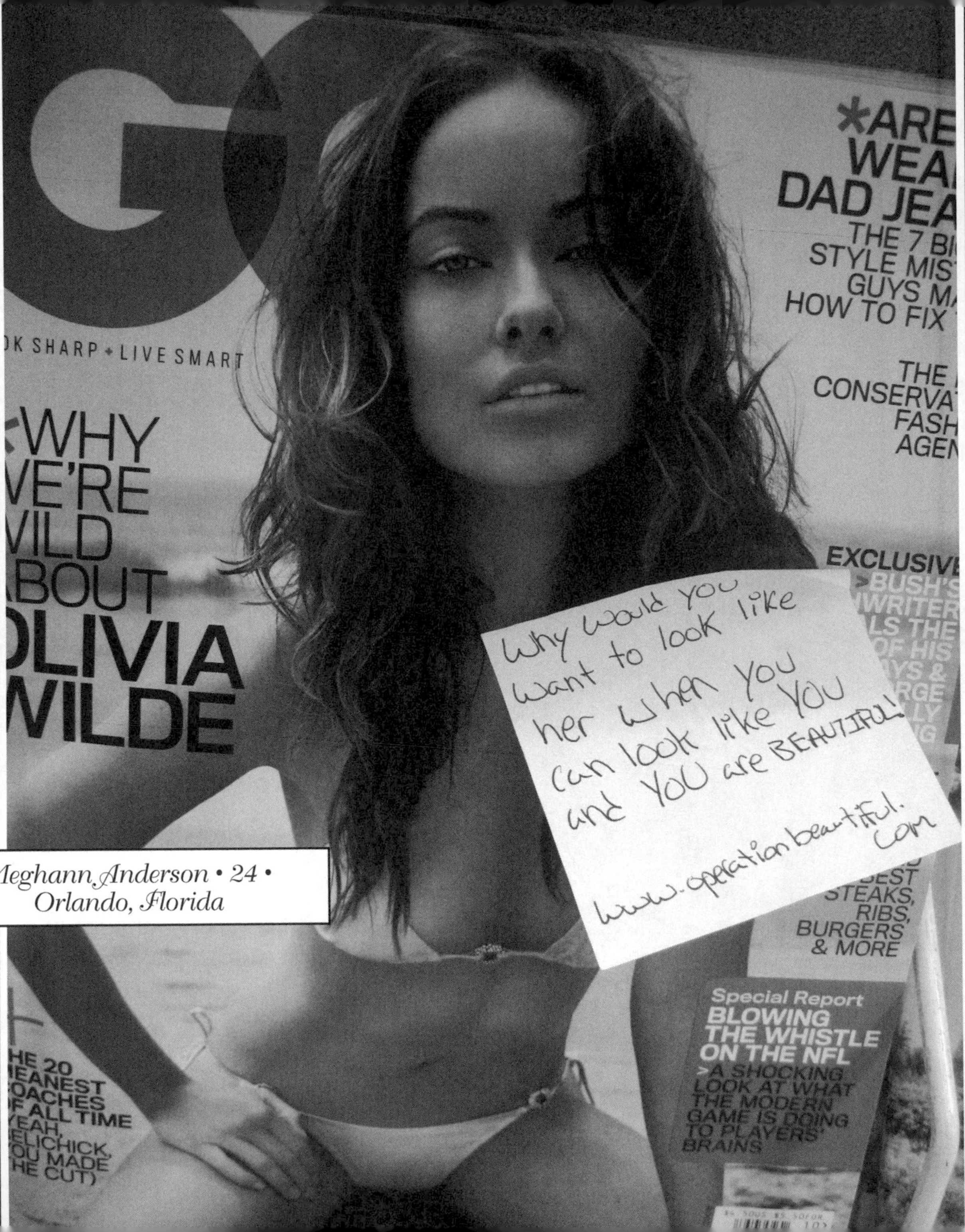

Meghann Anderson • 24 •
Orlando, Florida

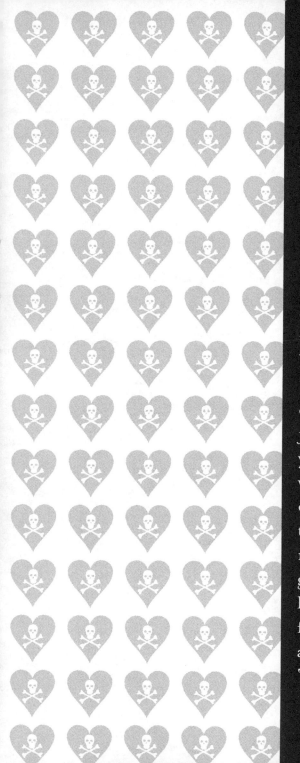

"I was struggling with an eating disorder and after a day filled with tears and hopelessness, one of my closest friends suggested I start writing down three positive things about myself each day. She said, 'I know it's hard right now, but try.' So I started writing each day, for months. There were countless pages I scribbled over, pages I ripped up, and journals I threw out. But I did write down three things every day. Sometimes they were the same three things, and sometimes they were things I barely believed.

During that time, my dad said to me, 'I don't understand it. You, of all people, don't judge anyone. Yet, you are so hard on yourself.' I started to wonder if this was how I wanted to live the rest of my life—unhappy, exhausted, and chasing a dream (perfection) that doesn't exist. One day, I woke up and realized I just wanted to be happy. I wanted to go out with my friends and not secretly be having anxiety about what I was going to order for dinner. I wanted to put on a new outfit and think, 'Hey, I look pretty hot!' and not 'My thighs are too big.' Basically, I wanted to be in the moment. I wanted to LIVE and not just survive. So many women say they're on a diet. When I was in the depths of my eating disorder, I wasn't on a food diet. I was on a diet from life!

I have learned that imperfections are what make me who I am. I love my blue eyes, the freckle on my left hand, and how cute my toes look after a pedicure. I love how free I feel when I put on my sweatpants after a long day and dance around the room. And I love how good it feels to be able to just breathe—to be me—and to accept who I am.

Our society brainwashes us with what the ideal woman 'should' look like. But it's time to tell ourselves positive messages."

Nicole Getman • 26 • Buffalo, New York

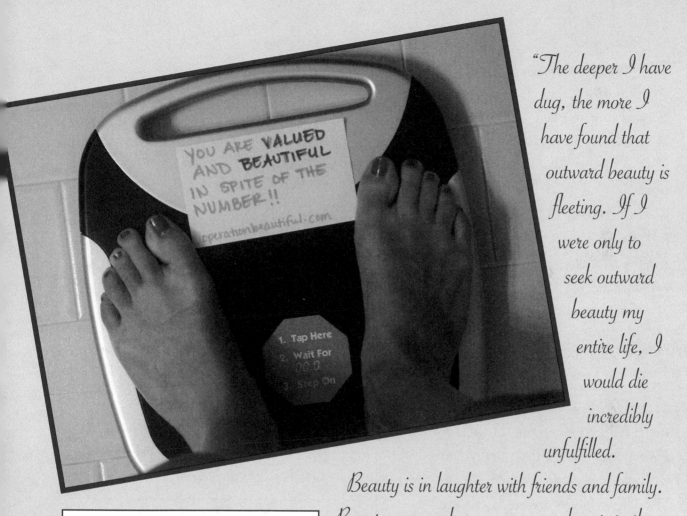

Jessica Daly • 24 • Trexlertown, Pennsylvania

"The deeper I have dug, the more I have found that outward beauty is fleeting. If I were only to seek outward beauty my entire life, I would die incredibly unfulfilled. Beauty is in laughter with friends and family. Beauty comes when we open our hearts to those in need. Beauty is watching the sunrise on your back porch with your spouse. Beauty is in me. Beauty is not skin deep."

"I have spent my entire life struggling with a healthy body. While my mom is the main person telling me not everyone is meant to be a size two, that is just what she is. Both my mother and my two sisters, one a year older than me, the other a year younger, are very petite. My stepmom says that outward appearances shouldn't matter, but she always downgrades herself and has undergone three different forms of plastic surgery, plus a breast augmentation. I'm working on finding my own healthy perspective."

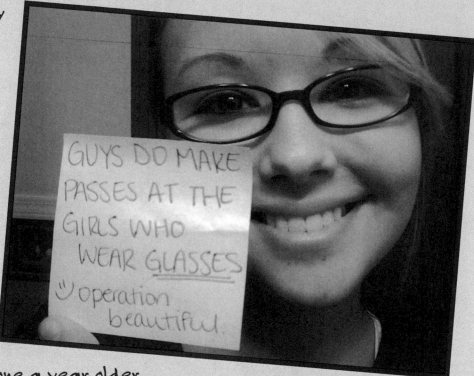

Jessica Y. • 20 • Beaumont, Texas

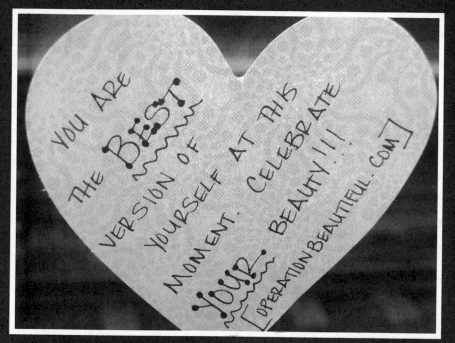

"When I was in high school, I was emotionally abusive to myself. Strangers, some friends, and even family would comment on my weight, and my body image fell apart. I was convinced that if I lost weight, I would be more attractive and could change how the world perceived me. I ate very little and worked out two hours a day, seven days a week. The only person I was kidding was myself. Now I'm twenty-four years old and on the verge of my twenty-fifth birthday. I'm in the most stable relationship of my life and love who I am. After years of battling weight and seeking therapy for my struggles, I have come to love me. But it wasn't until a few months ago, when I heard about Operation Beautiful through a family member, that I really started to advocate for **real** beauty and myself."

Lauren • 24 • Perkasie, Pennsylvania

Your Own Beauty

It's time to let go of society's Thin Ideal and create your own concept of beauty. Change how you see, not how you look!

- Be critical of how beauty is presented by the media. The vast majority of photographs in fashion and entertainment magazines have been digitally altered—legs lengthened, thighs trimmed, and waists shrunk. Do you realize the hair in shampoo commercials is computer generated? Inspect advertisements or magazine covers and ask yourself if the image is realistic. "Women who regularly compare their bodies to the falseness of these images tend to have the worst personal body image," says Dr. Martz.

- Be the best version of yourself right now. Instead of focusing on the person you have been or the person you could be, relish the wonderful characteristics you already have. Life is far too short to waste your energy focusing on anything besides the present.

- Take pride in your physical appearance, no matter what your size, age, look, or shape. It can feel so wonderful to wear a flattering shirt, a beautiful necklace, or a killer pair of heels! Take the time to

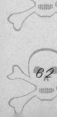
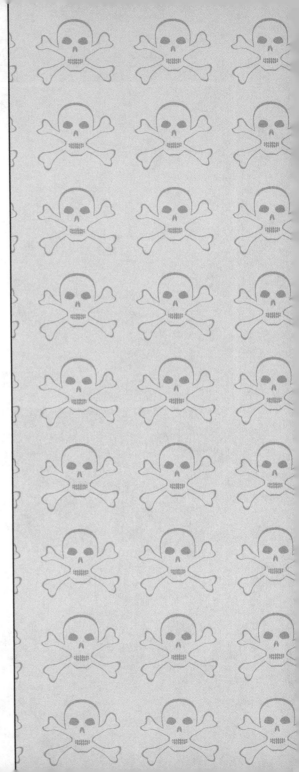

choose outfits that make you feel special or treat yourself to small pleasures, like facials or manicures. This is about defining your own version of beautiful and celebrating your body, not about conforming to the unrealistic and impossibly strict standards of the Thin Ideal.

- Stop calorie counting and start living! Your body is so valuable—it allows you to experience many amazing things that most of us take for granted. Focus on the fact that you can run, dance, smile, sing, kiss, and laugh.

- Work out to feel strong and healthy, not to be skinny. Try challenging yourself to set new fitness goals that have nothing to do with your size; for example, train to do ten push-ups in a row or swim 1,600 meters without stopping.

- Nourish your body with healthy food and balanced portions. Focus on your long-term health goals instead of your weight.

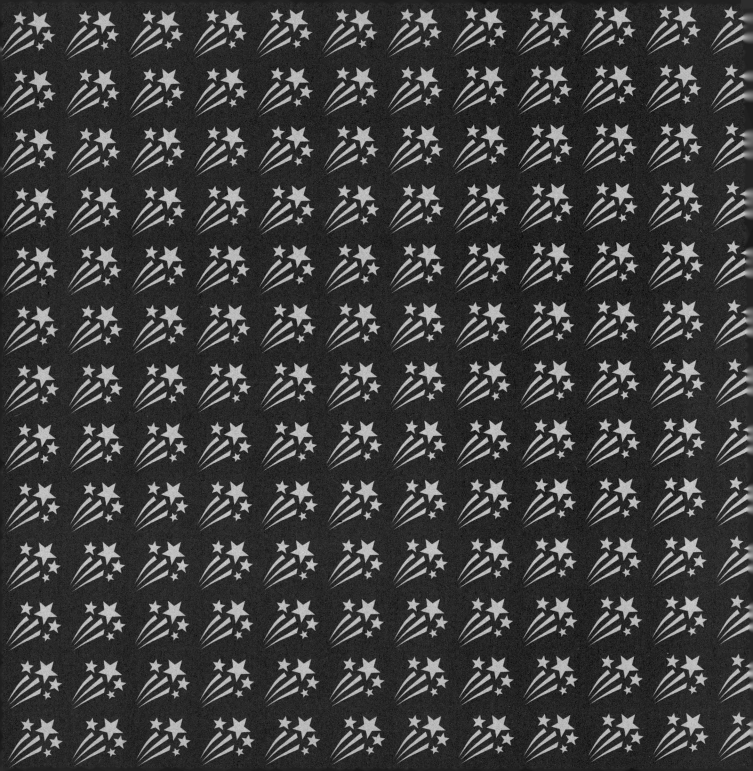

Chapter 3

Family and Friends

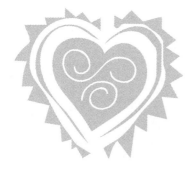

An Outside Influence

*I*magine yourself standing naked in front of a mirror. Don't shy away from the image. Just observe your body, without criticism and without timidity. Run your eyes across your arms and chest, down your stomach, and along your legs. Inspect your freckles or wrinkles, your teeth, the way your face is not perfectly symmetrical. Find the unique parts that distinguish your body from someone else's. The scars, the bumps, the cellulite, the muscles . . . take it all in. This is your body, and it's the only one you'll ever have.

When you are not consciously separating emotion from your body image, how do you see yourself? What feelings wash over you when you peer into the mirror? For so many girls and women, their mental picture of their body is intrinsically wrapped up in things that have nothing to do with their physical appearance. We "wear" so many experiences on our body image—

> *This is your body, and it's the only one you'll ever have.*

emotions associated with that extra slice of cake at dinner last night, our relationships, the extra mile we ran at the gym, our childhoods, and the satisfaction we receive from our job or schoolwork. Our body image reflects much more than our appearance. It reflects how we feel about our lives in general.

Perhaps the strongest outside influence on our self-image is the relationships we have with our family members and friends. Whether positive or negative, the experiences with the people close to us can shape our self-confidence, our outlook, and the respect we give to ourselves. The mission of Operation Beautiful extends far beyond encouraging women to stop Fat Talking. Operation Beautiful is about loving and respecting ourselves fully, which allows us to become more open to forming healthy, compassionate relationships with the other beautiful people in our lives.

Very few people are blessed with fulfilling relationships with *every* person in their lives. But every single one of us has a choice to interact and react to the people we know in a healthy way. We have a choice to nurture positive relationships and disengage from negative ones. We have a choice to support people who support us. We can decide to raise our children differently than we were raised, and we can select an encouraging and caring partner to share our lives with, if we wish. Most importantly, we can choose to be proactive in the development of our self-worth, and we can use all our experiences with family and friends to create a deeper understanding about life, love, and true happiness.

Like most people, Deb's parents had a profound impact on her self-esteem while she was growing up. "They were very supportive, and I believed they boosted my self-esteem,"

remembers Deb, who is forty-four years old and lives in Southern California. "I was always encouraged to try various activities and continue with those I liked." Despite her parents' best efforts, Deb eventually found herself ninety pounds overweight. "I went on my first Atkins diet with my mom," she recalls. "She dieted hard and often."

Tired of crash dieting without long-term success, Deb adopted a more balanced and maintainable approach to eating and exercise, and she lost the weight. Sadly, her mother developed multiple sclerosis, and she continued to put on weight as her body failed. "Toward the end of life, my mom's only pleasures were television and food. I never, ever suggested she try to lose weight," Deb sighs. "In fact, she was the one bothered by it, and the week before she died, she told me she was going to go back on Atkins after the holidays." The gravity of her mother's "lifelong yo-yo dieting habits" had a profound impact on Deb's self-image. "When I think about the fact that she was worried about losing weight and only had a week to live—it makes me want to never obsess about food and body-image issues," says Deb. "I just want to be healthy and balanced."

Deb's father is also struggling with a serious illness—Non-Hodgkin's lymphoma—and she accompanies him to doctors' appointments and social outings. "It's a shame, but it was his illness that brought us closer," she says. "After spending so many hours together while my dad has been in treatment, we have discovered that we have a deep friendship. We confide in each other, and he supports me as much as I support him." To pass time at the hospital, Deb frequently finds herself wandering the halls, posting Operation Beautiful notes in bathrooms, on signs, in the gift shop, and inside magazines in the waiting room. "We see men and women of all ages in the cancer treatment center," says Deb. "I've seen young women with no hair from chemotherapy, and I know that must hit them hard. If I was in that situation, I would think finding a note would make me happier. Hopefully, these messages are internalized."

Deb's experiences with her mother and father have profoundly impacted the way she views her health, not just her pant size, as staying healthy is one of the biggest priorities in Deb's life. Deb strives to eat wholesome, natural foods, and she says exercise helps her relieve stress. "Sometimes I'm in kickboxing class and when they call for a really vicious kick or punch, I imagine that I'm obliterating multiple sclerosis, leukemia, or lymphoma," Deb says. "Once my workout is done, I can give more of myself to others for the rest of the day. If I skip my workout, I have less to give others. I see it like the analogy of the oxygen mask on a plane: Put on your mask before assisting others. Same thing with exercise—it's my oxygen. I literally need it to breathe."

Blood Draw

You are lovely just the way you are ♡ operationbeautiful.com

Cancer cannot take away your inner beauty. www.operationbeautiful.com

Deb • 44 • California

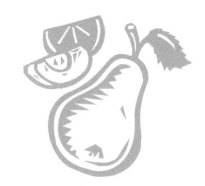

"For my friend Ibelis's birthday, I bought her a load of Post-it notes and wrote her an Operation Beautiful note. A few weeks later, we set up a date to go on an Operation Beautiful spree! We went to a few locations to post the notes, and everywhere we looked, it seemed like Operation Beautiful was needed! At first, we were nervous about people seeing us and tried to hide what we were doing. By the end of the day, we were sticking them right on magazines in the crowded checkout lane. We realized we didn't care who saw us or what they thought——we had nothing to be ashamed of because we were spreading a beautiful message!"

Ali • 26 • Boston, Massachusetts

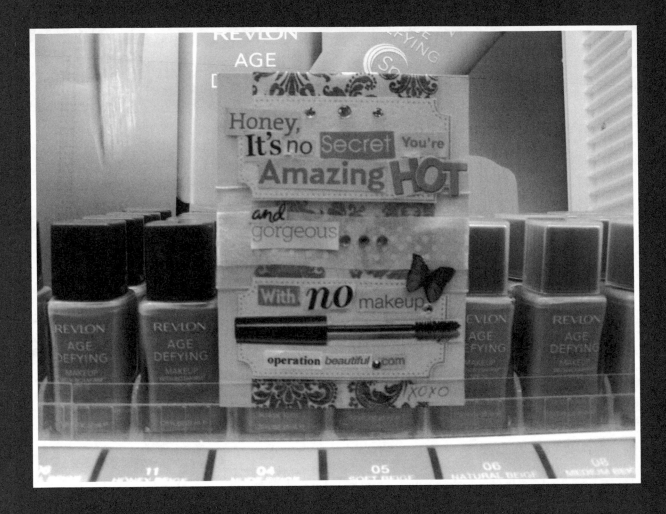

"I grew up in a Pentecostal church where women choose not to wear cosmetics. During my first year in college, I started to become more independent from the church, and for the first time, I experimented with makeup. Wearing a little mascara and lip gloss was fun, and I liked the feeling of getting all girly. As time has gone by I found myself with not just a little lip gloss, but a full face of makeup.

My daily routine to get ready consisted of applying foundation, concealer, bronzer, blush, lipstick, eyeliner, eye shadow, and three coats of mascara. While living with my boyfriend, I would sleep in my makeup so the next morning he wouldn't see me without it. I wouldn't even think about working out at the gym without it. Hollywood and magazines filled with beautiful women with painted lips and perfect faces reminded me that I looked pale and plain without cosmetics.

My views on beauty changed when my baby niece was born into this world. Baby Emery is absolutely gorgeous. All babies are 100 percent natural beauties. No one would dare cover up or try to change their dainty, pretty features. So, why do things change when we become young women? We are wrongfully pressured to camouflage and modify the natural beauty that we were brought into this world with. This made me realize that I need to stop obsessing about concealing my chicken pox scars and freckles and contouring my potato nose.

I still wear makeup, but I don't cake it on anymore. I went through my cosmetics and threw away a large portion of my collection. Today, I'm not afraid to go to the gym without makeup, and I even let my boyfriend see me without it. I wanted to remind women that they are beautiful naturally, so I left a little piece of encouragement in the cosmetics department at my local Target."

Janae Trujillo • 24 • Denver, Colorado

"My mom is suffering from stage 3 colon cancer. For the past eight months, she has been doing chemotherapy four days a week and just finished her last session. I took my mom out to dinner and a movie to celebrate her last round of chemotherapy, and during dinner I told her that she looked beautiful. She responded by saying, 'I don't feel very beautiful' and described how she felt that the chemotherapy made her look old—her skin is dry, her nose is all sore (from constantly bleeding), and her hair has gotten very thin. I have noticed all of these things, but I still feel like she is the most beautiful woman in the world, and I wanted to let her know that. I left her this note, as well as another one to post on the bathroom mirror the next time she goes to the cancer center for a checkup."

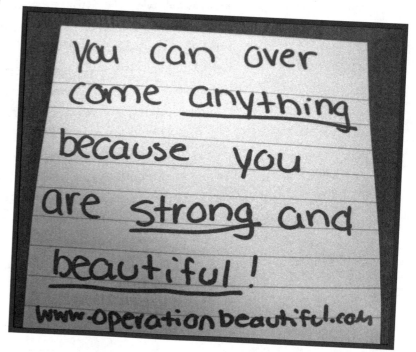

Megan M. • 24 • Middletown, New Jersey

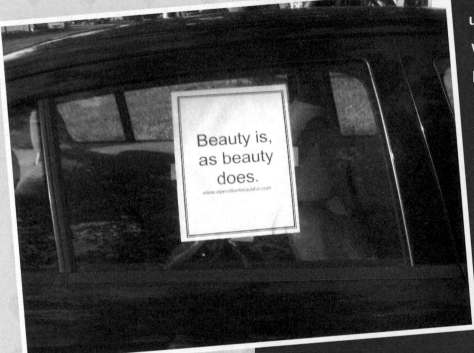

"While I was growing up, I never felt like I was good enough or pretty enough. As I get older, I see that beauty is so much more than that. I decided to place this Operation Beautiful note on my car window. This way, men can see the message, too! Ever since I've put up the note on the side of my car, I've gotten my fair share of honks and waves. It's good to be noticed for spreading hope and beauty! I hope that everyone who sees my car goes home and tells their families and friends about Operation Beautiful."

Danielle VanMarter • 21 • Niagara Falls, New York

"I am the activity director at Parkview, an independent living facility in Knoxville, Tennessee. After checking out the Operation Beautiful site on the computer, it gave me an idea to do a special project with the residents. I asked the residents their thoughts on beauty, and we posted the notes on our bulletin boards. It was great fun, and it allowed us to have an open conversation about what real beauty means. It was interesting to hear the perspective of people who have lived long lives and have experience and wisdom behind them."

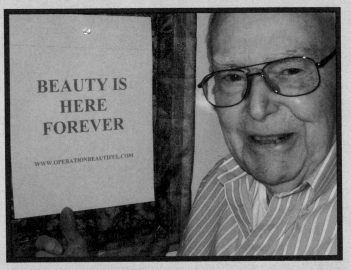

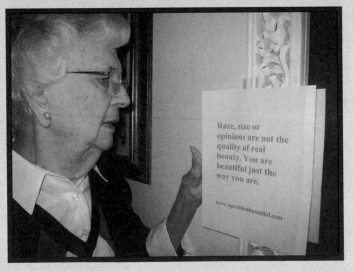

Cherie Meece • 50 • Powell, Tennessee

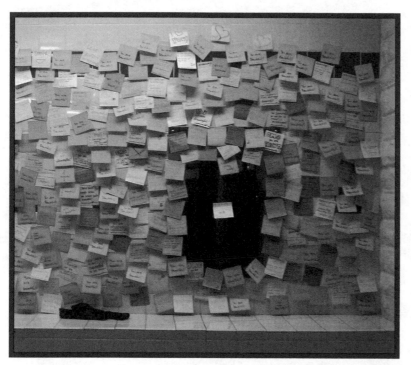

"We woke up early to get to school at six A.M. We covered the two mirrors in the main bathroom on campus with notes that said 'You are beautiful!' and encouraged the girls to take whatever note they liked the most. We continually went into the bathroom to check on the status of the mirrors, and every time, there was a crowd of girls surrounding the mirrors, reading and picking out their favorite note. One of my other friends said she saw one girl just glance at the mirror with a huge grin on her face. Every time we walked out of the bathroom, we had one on our faces, too! We are so happy of the outcome of the Operation Beautiful attack that we're planning a bigger one—we're going to put notes surrounding every mirror in the school and entirely cover the wall in the main bathroom!"

Emily M. and Kailey S. • 17 • Fullerton, California

"I was diagnosed with breast cancer this past summer. My daughter stayed by my side through my bilateral mastectomy and reconstructive surgery. Every hospital visit, she left Operation Beautiful notes in magazines, on calendars, and in breast cancer information books in the exam rooms. I eventually received an Operation Beautiful note from my daughter in the mail! I keep it on the fridge now, and it never fails to make me smile."

Julie A. • 47 • Camp Lejeune,
North Carolina

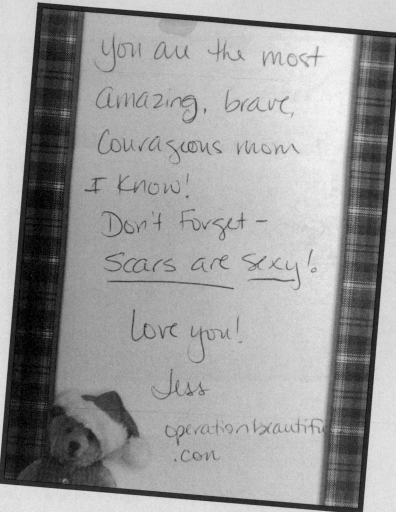

You are the most amazing, brave, courageous mom I know! Don't forget — Scars are sexy! Love you! Jess operationbeautiful.com

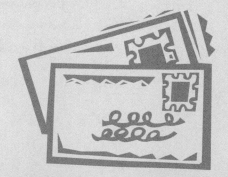

Doris • 67 • Sacramento, California

"As a shut-in with a disability, I felt left out of Operation Beautiful. I thought the idea was inspired, but didn't see any way for me to leave messages because I rarely leave the house. Then, I decided to add it to my signature line on my e-mails to my friends. Now my signature reads, 'Beauty is in the eye of the beholder. Be the beholder. www.operationbeautiful.com'!"

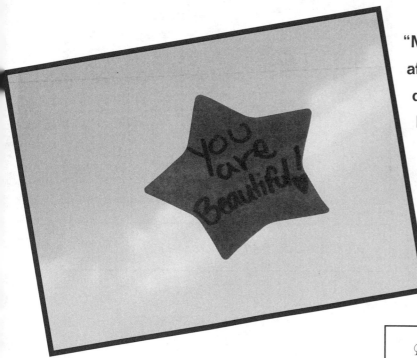

"My sister and I are very close. But after a year at college together, we decided to go to different schools. I feel like a part of me is missing, and it's hard not having her here. Whenever I think of my note, I think of Heather and how beautiful we are as sisters. Every day, I thank Jesus for the wonderful sister He gave me."

Penny • 20 • Oak Hills, California

"I took my two young daughters to the library. I grabbed a pack of notes and a marker, planning to leave a note on the mirror of the children's restroom and in books, knowing that it would be seen by other mothers of small children, like myself. At the library, I pulled a copy of *Fit From Within* off the shelf, a book that helped me learn to truly accept myself and love myself for who I was. When I put the note in the book, my five-year-old was watching me and asked what it said. I told her, 'You are beautiful.' When she asked who was beautiful, I hugged her close and said, 'You are!'"

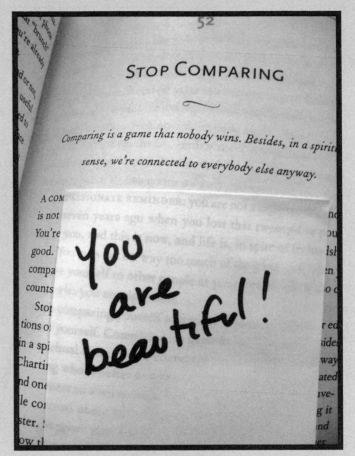

Alison Spath • 30 • Rochester, New York

THE POSITIVE PEOPLE

Do you know someone who always makes you laugh, who values your opinion, and who believes you can achieve your dreams? If you're having a bad day, do you always call the same person? Our support team—our Positive People—encourages us to live our best life. Some people know just one Positive Person, and others are blessed with many Positive People on their side.

Our worth is not determined by others; however, our friends and family are the strongest outside influence on our self-image. That is why it's pivotal that we identify and nurture the healthy relationships in our lives.

Our interactions with Positive People are not always perfect—miscommunications, the little hassles of everyday life, and other heartaches can erode the trust between two people. Imagine that your life is a garden, and the Positive People you know are beautiful flowers. To keep your garden strong and healthy, you must tend to your flowers and snip away any weeds.

Here are some simple steps to nurture the relationships with the Positive People in your life:

- Emotions are contagious. Believe that you are worthy of love and support from Positive People in your life, and it will be so. Similarly, give respect to your Positive People, and they will feel more respect for themselves.

- Frequently tell your Positive People how much you appreciate their support—don't assume they know the amazing impact they have on your life! Never underestimate the power of a quick phone call, e-mail, or Operation Beautiful note.

- When a personal disaster strikes a Positive Person in your life, allow your Positive Person to lead the conversation. Refrain from "explaining away" or "solving" their grief or anger.

- Even between two Positive People, advice can be tricky. When you give unsolicited advice, it can seem as if you are imposing your beliefs. Practice the act of listening as opposed to mindless chatter when a friend comes to you with a concern.

- Make exciting memories with your Positive People. Sign up for a 5K race, enroll in a baking class, or try indoor rock climbing together.

- Do not rely on your Positive People to make you happy. True happiness comes from within, and when we look toward other people for happiness, we are setting ourselves up for failure. The Positive People in our lives should enrich us, teach us, and love us, but at the end of the day, our happiness is our own responsibility. This mind-set allows us to have a mutually supportive relationship with the Positive People in our lives.

Energy Vampires and Negative Noise

"Our entire team was terrified of our boss, who was aggressive and unsupportive. It created such a tense work environment," recalls Anne P. of Washington, D.C. The breaking point came when Anne developed a painful migraine in the middle of the workday, and her boss refused to let her leave. "I didn't even know what to say to her, so I just turned on my heel, went to the bathroom, and cried. It was horrible. I had no idea why someone would be so cold and cruel," Anne says.

She soon realized that the only way to deal with her boss was to let the mean comments slide. "I told myself that there must be some reason she was so miserable. She was obviously very unhappy and tried to make others that way, too," says Anne, who soon found another job. "My boss was a major Energy Vampire."

Energy Vampires are negative people who leave us feeling emotionally exhausted after interacting with them. These soul-suckers use backhanded compliments to make us feel small. Energy Vampires may be highly passive-aggressive and engage in subtle criticism or guilt. Energy Vampires drain us of our positivity through hostility, manipulation, or neediness.

Energy Vampires speak a language known as Negative Noise. Negative Noise is upsetting and distracting, and it can deflate your confidence or mood. An Energy Vampire may say, "You are so lucky you can eat so much food! I would get really fat!" or "My job is *so* demanding and hard, and everyone depends on me! You must love your easy job." This Negative Noise can overwhelm all the positive encouragement in your life.

Anne was lucky in the sense that her Energy Vampire was her boss. Anne could choose to find a new job and eliminate the Negative Noise from her life. But Energy Vampires come in all forms—as parents, children, sisters, brothers, friends, and lovers—and it's not always possible or easy to walk away.

"My mother is a little black hole, sucking everything into a negative space within her," says Angi, a twenty-six-year-old Canadian. In a misplaced attempt to deal with the pressure from her mother, Angi developed an eating disorder. "But now I lift weights, box, and practice Tai Chi to get rid of negative energy/thoughts around me. It focuses my mind and blanks out all that craziness. I also post Operation Beautiful notes from time to time!"

Like Angi, Jessica's Energy Vampires were lurking in her own family. "When I was growing up, my mom and grandmother always called me fat and used Fat Talk. I have lived with that in my head for years now, and I

Angi • 26 • *St. Catharines, Ontario, Canada*

am finally learning to put it to rest," says Jessica, who is twenty-seven and lives in South Carolina. "I made a deal with myself that I will not let what others say tear me down anymore. I am who I am and I am happy with me."

Linzi Bommarito of Boise, Idaho, encountered an Energy Vampire when she asked a friend to be her workout buddy. "At first, it was great. We went to the gym together a few times," says Linzi. "But then she would ask me to have a wine night instead of a workout. Or she would promise to meet me at the gym and bail at the last minute." Linzi eventually decided she couldn't rely on her friend to help guide her to a healthier lifestyle. "I was sabotaging myself by hanging out with temptation. My friend wasn't a bad person, but we were just in different places. We have similar goals, but she isn't yet ready to put in the work."

The ultimate antidote to Energy Vampires and Negative Noise is positivity. "We only become victims of vampires if we let ourselves," points out Sarah Matheny, a thirty-one-year-old mother of two young daughters. "I could sit and cry about the fact that I don't have the perfect mother, in-law, sibling, friend, or whoever that responds with positive feedback, love, and support. On the other hand, I can put that aside and accept that being negative is their problem. This allows me to focus my efforts on being the best mother, wife, friend, and person that I can be, so that ultimately I don't become an Energy Vampire myself."

"I always wanted to post an Operation Beautiful note at my school. One day, after fitness class, I was changing in the locker room and could overhear all these negative comments, such as 'Look how fat I am' or 'I am so ugly.' It made me so sad. I posted this note on the mirror, hoping—and kind of knowing—that it would touch some of my peers and stop the body bashing. It's still up there (a whole week later!) and I haven't heard any hateful remarks since!"

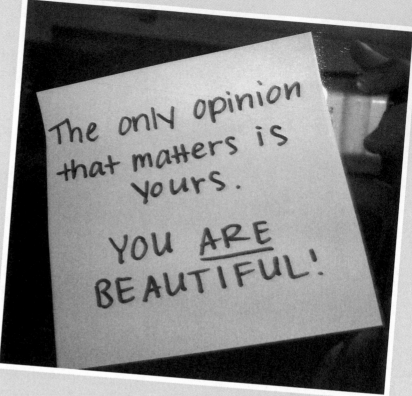

The only opinion that matters is yours.

YOU ARE BEAUTIFUL!

Laura E. • 16 • Nebraska

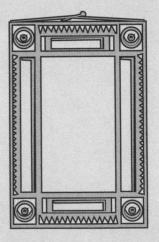

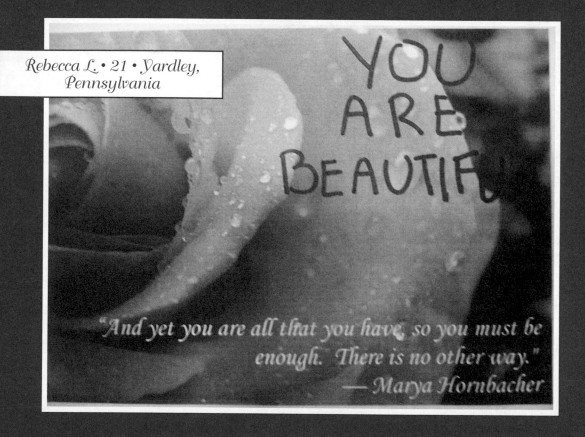

Rebecca L. • 21 • Yardley, Pennsylvania

YOU ARE BEAUTIFUL

"And yet you are all that you have, so you must be enough. There is no other way."
— Marya Hornbacher

"I believe in the power of kindness and the impact of one person's mood on another's, like a domino effect. I was an inpatient at Princeton University Medical Center's Eating Disorder Unit. One Friday night I noticed the mood of the girls on the unit was extremely low and negative. I decided to take action. I bought a single rose for each girl, attached this note, and left it at each chair in the dining room. I cannot put into words how surprised, grateful, and loved each and every girl felt the moment they walked in the room and found their individual rose."

"For as long as I can remember, my mom has been obsessed about <u>my</u> weight. She would call me fat to my face and make me weigh myself weekly, in front of her. It got to the point where I would weigh myself five or six times a day as well. It destroyed my self-confidence and inhibited my sense of reality. I stumbled upon the Operation Beautiful site in the summer, and the notes posted made me cry. I felt like they were screaming my name, written just for me. Soon after, I left home for college and everything changed. This place is filled with love and acceptance. I love myself and look into the mirror and see the gorgeous, loving, crazy girl that I always was."

Megzee • 19 • St. Louis, Missouri

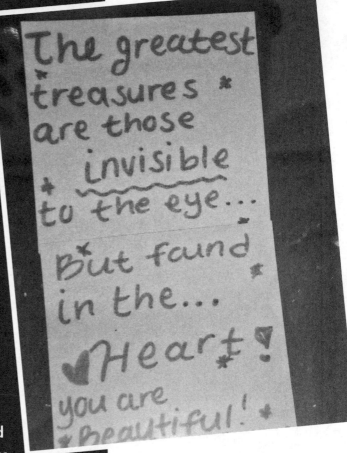

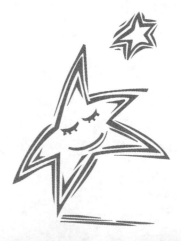

88

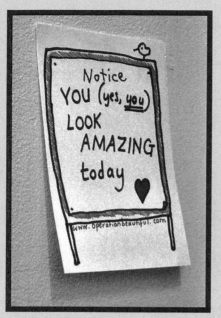

"*I was bullied quite nastily throughout high school, and to have read a note like this on the girls' bathroom mirror or to have been told this by someone would've really made my day. Something small can be so powerful.*"

Elizabeth • 18 • West Midlands,
United Kingdom

"Nothing is worse than thinking you are not good enough. I gave this note to a dear friend who had just moved to New York and is in a low spot in her life. In a new place, she has no close friends and boy problems. I sent her this note in hopes she understands that she is beautiful—she really is."

Tasha K. • 26 • Seattle, Washington

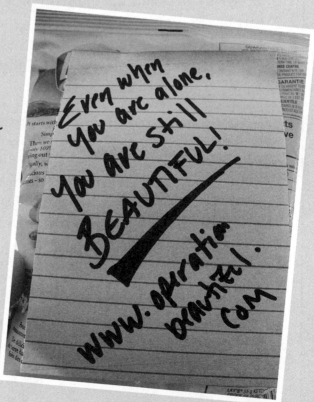

Shut Out Energy Vampires

- Energy Vampires feed off your reaction to their Negative Noise, so ignore the behavior as much as possible. Instead of getting upset, use a visualization trick to help the comments roll right off you. "It sounds silly, but whenever I'm in a situation when someone is spewing negativity either at me or around me, I sort of pretend I have on a yellow raincoat," says Michele, a thirty-five-year-old from Ohio. "I think of their words and negativity like rain hitting the yellow rain slicker—the waterproof coat doesn't let it inside to get me wet—the negativity flows away, leaving me grounded in peace and pleasantness!"

- Consider the many reasons why the person might be so negative, and turn your anger into sympathetic detachment. With sympathetic detachment, you can understand the motivations behind their Negative Noise and recognize that it has very little to do with you personally.

- Understand that your Energy Vampire may be projecting his or her own negative self-image onto you. "When people criticize you for your weight or other things, consider that it is often a direct reflection of how they feel about themselves, rather than a truth about you," says Dr. Susan Albers, a

psychologist who specializes in relationship and weight issues.

- Focus on something upbeat. "Working in the concert industry, I have experienced my fair share of Energy Vampires due to crazy deadlines and constant pressure. To relax, I listen to music," says Laura M., a twenty-seven-year-old from Milwaukee. "In my iTunes, the most played track is 'Wouldn't It Be Nice' by the Beach Boys. Listening to upbeat, positive music keeps things in perspective, and I feel like I am capable of whatever is thrown at me!"

- Disengage yourself from the situation. You have a right to remove yourself from toxic workplaces or relationships. It can be difficult to fully disengage from family members or friends, so consider limiting your discussions to non-confrontational topics.

- Similarly, choose to spend your time wisely. Instead of wasting your energy dealing with a soul-sucking Energy Vampire, call up an old friend, post an Operation Beautiful note, or do something nice for a stranger.

- Remember that an Energy Vampire only has control over you if you let them. While you can't control others' actions, you can control how you react to a situation.

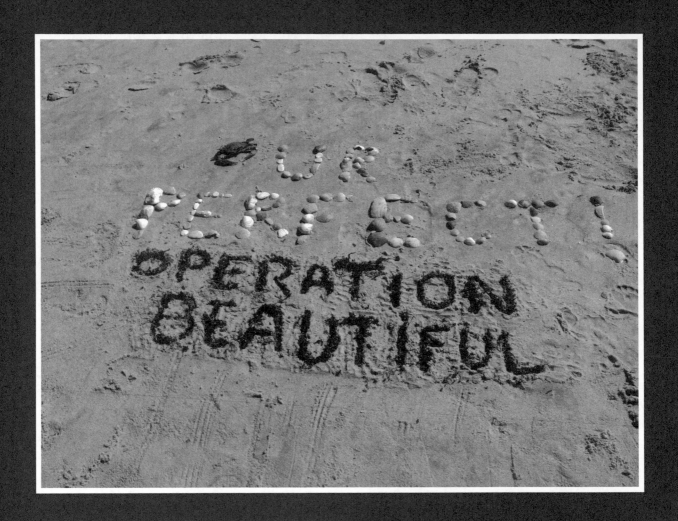

Sarah Eamigh • 25 • Winchester, Virginia

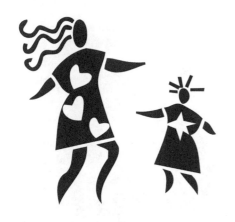

Starting the Conversation

Whether children will grow up practicing positive or negative habits is greatly influenced by their parents, older siblings, aunts, teachers, coaches, and other role models. In fact, toxic habits such as Fat Talk are often profoundly ingrained behaviors learned over many years, even stretching as far back as childhood. "Kids absorb every single word," says Dr. Albers, who notes that we must be aware of how our body image issues impact the younger generation of both boys and girls.

Carla Birnberg, a former personal trainer who has competed in fitness and bodybuilding competitions, says that "few things are more important to me than raising a happy, healthy daughter who is 100 percent comfortable in her own skin." Her three-year-old daughter, Emma-Louise, is a curious little girl with a big smile and dark brown eyes who frequently sports a T-shirt with the words *I Heart Myself* embossed on the front.

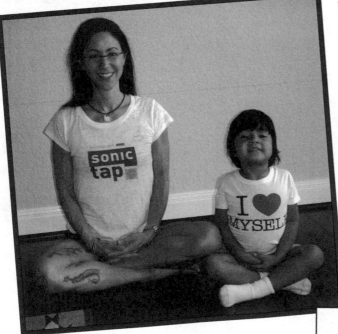

Carla Birnberg • 40 • Austin, Texas

"In my opinion, we need to start talking about self-love as soon as our daughters can hear us," she says. Carla admits that it can be difficult to find a way to start the conversation, especially with younger children, which is why she took Emma-Louise on an Operation Beautiful note-posting spree.

"I resisted the urge to launch into a tirade about makeup and women feeling pressure to wear it in order to be seen as beautiful, the media's standardized image of beauty, and women feeling pressure to be skinny," Carla says. "Parenthood, to me, has been a learning curve of listening to what she is really asking, hearing her, and answering that specific question."

To explain the Operation Beautiful concept, Carla used an analogy of a playground bully. After all, to a toddler, everyone seems quite wonderful, unless they push you into the dirt or steal the ball. Carla used this concept to explain to Emma-Louise that beauty comes from the inside.

Carla and Emma-Louise posted notes in changing rooms, on cars, and on the scale at the gym. Since Emma-Louise is so young, Carla wrote the notes herself but asked her daughter for suggestions and

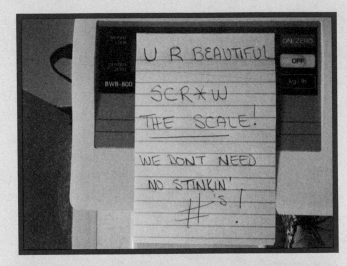

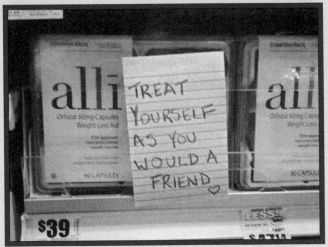

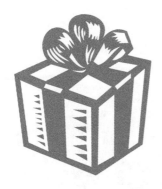

talked about the meaning of each note. Emma-Louise enjoyed the mission more than Carla ever dreamed possible. "I can tell she got the point of Operation Beautiful in her own way by how she's behaved since that day," Carla says. "I've watched her make time to say nice things to friends and strangers in a way she didn't before."

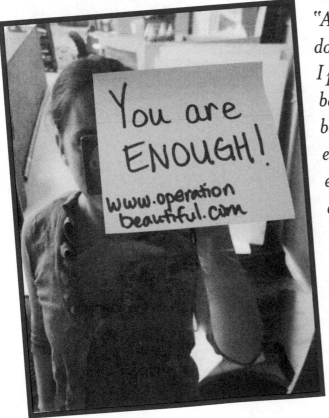

You are ENOUGH!

www.operation beautiful.com

"As a teacher, I try to push students to do their best work and be their best selves. I posted this note in the high school bathroom. It's meant for the girls who never believe they are smart, pretty, or skinny enough. It's so important for girls everywhere to know that they are good enough and can achieve great things."

Heather Pare • 29 • Glen Ridge, New Jersey

"All through elementary school, my parents read me Dr. Seuss books before bed, and I have to admit that it made me somewhat of an overly-obsessed Whoville fan! My infatuation with all things Dr. Seuss, however, did some good during my freshman year of college. All the girls in my dorm room were feeling sub-par due to the 'thin-is-better' mentality of college girls in general. With a couple other friends, I left notes like this one in classrooms, written on index cards and taped to the desks. How could someone's day not be brighter after reading this cute quote?"

Gelsey K. • *19* • *Richmond, Virginia*

Today you are You, that is truer than true. There is no one alive who is Youer than You!

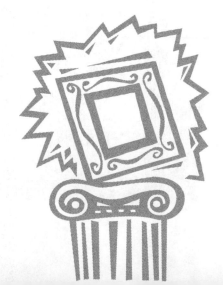

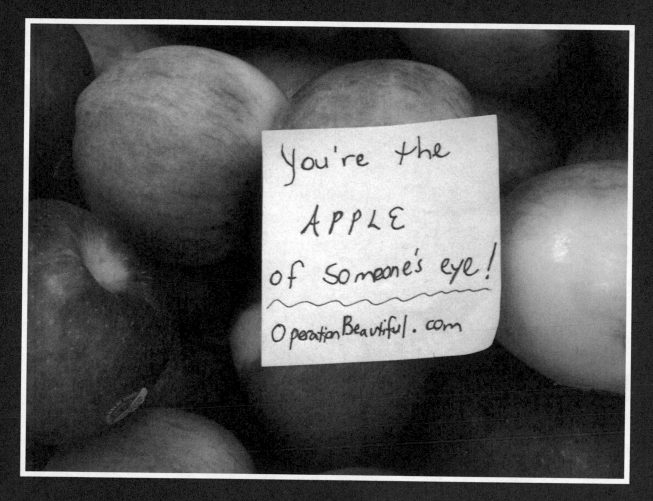

You're the
APPLE
of someone's eye!

OperationBeautiful.com

"During my childhood, I never thought I was very pretty. I saw all my flaws and imperfections and believed I was ugly. However, my mother would always tell me, 'You are the apple of my eye, and you are beautiful.' Secretly, I thought, 'You're

Jana • 46 • Garland, Texas

supposed to say that——you're my mom.' My mom passed away almost eighteen years ago now, and one of the main things I remember about her is the many positive messages I heard from her. I still have those same 'flaws and imperfections,' but I often remind myself of what my mother told me over and over while I was growing up . . . and now I actually believe it! This is testament to how very important our words are to other people. We really do start to believe the messages we hear from people——all the more reason to make those messages positive!"

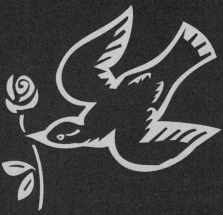

"Having to be both parents when my husband is deployed is a challenge. Even more so given that both of our children are boys, and they miss having a male role model so much of the time. My oldest son, who's six years old, and I went on a mom and son 'date' recently. I knew it would be the perfect opportunity to share the Operation Beautiful message with him and others. He asked about the notes we posted, and I told him that it's nice to do something for people, even if it's for strangers, and even if they don't know who did it for them. He has come to understand that if Mommy is having a rough day, she'll often post notes because it makes her feel better to do something for others."

Samantha S. • 31 • Santa Rita, Guam

"*I put this note right beside a baby changing station in the Charlotte Douglas International Airport. I saw several women with babies rushing off to a flight with a baby in their arms and a big baby bag. It didn't look easy! I know I would be frazzled, so I thought a little note of encouragement might brighten their day. Being a mom is hard work. We shouldn't forget to stop and let new moms know they are doing a good job and they're beautiful.*"

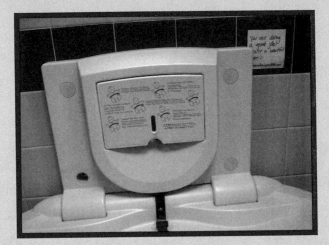

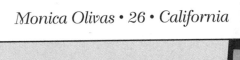

Monica Olivas • 26 • California

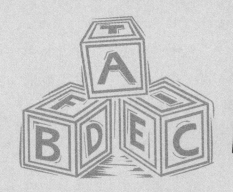

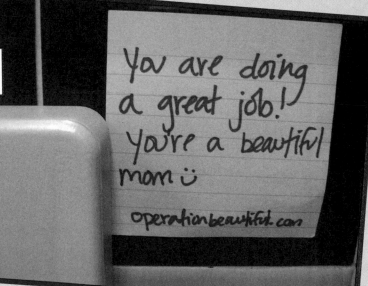

You are doing a great job! You're a beautiful mom :)

operationbeautiful.com

Raising Confident Children

Whether you're a mother, sister, babysitter, or coach, you can have a profound impact on the way a child views herself (or himself!). That's why we must stay conscious of the signals we send our children about body image and leading a positive lifestyle.

- It's never too early to start the conversation, but tailor discussions about body image to the child's age, as Carla did with Emma-Louise. With older girls, point out negative messages about body image in magazines or on television and ask for the child's opinion. If you see an obvious example of Photoshopping in an advertisement, for example, ask your daughter why she thinks the company did that and what the implications of that type of advertising are.

- "Be an unwavering role model," says Dr. Susan Albers. "Avoid Fat Talk or criticizing yourself, even on your very worst day. Additionally, communicate acceptance of your own body. Focus on what it does for you instead of what disappoints you about it." Tell your daughter you love and value yourself enough to treat yourself with kindness, no matter what.

- Compliment your daughters, emphasizing the qualities that make a person truly beautiful—kindness, generosity, moral fortitude, and other internal characteristics.

- If your daughter expresses concern about her appearance, listen to her carefully. Dismissing her fears at face value ("Don't be silly, your freckles aren't that noticeable!") stops the conversation dead in its tracks. She may have brought up the issue to discuss something else that is troubling her, such as an issue with school or a fight with a friend.

- Show your daughter that working out doesn't necessarily mean going to the gym. Play catch, go for a hike, or go for a bike ride after dinner. Let her choose the activity; after all, exercise should be fun!

- Empower your children by teaching them to choose and cook healthy, delicious foods. Declare one night a week "new recipe night," and work with your child to choose, shop for, and prepare the meal. "Children are more willing to try new foods or adopt healthy habits like exercising when they're involved in the process," says Janel Ovrut, a registered dietitian. "In addition, feeding your daughters nutritious foods that you won't eat yourself sends a strong negative message. Learn how to cook together so you can create healthy meals that you both enjoy and can learn from each other."

· Don't forget that boys struggle with body image, too. Young boys look to their idols—fast and lean quarterbacks and hunky leading men—and often wonder why they don't look the same way. Research has found that males comprise nearly 10 to 25 percent of anorexics and 40 percent of binge eaters. Emphasizing health and happiness to young boys is just as crucial as it is for girls.

· Ask your daughter or son to go on an Operation Beautiful date and spread positivity together!

Chapter 4

Fitness

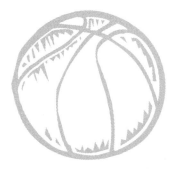

The Healthy Tipping Point

$\mathcal{A}$ normal shopping trip turned into a life-changing challenge for Annie, a sixteen-year-old from Minnesota. Annie and her father walked into the Ralph Lauren store, and when she spied an attractive polo shirt she thought he would like, she brought it over to him. "My dad looked at the shirt and said, 'I think I would have to lose thirty pounds to fit into anything in this store,'" remembers Annie. "He wasn't exactly a small person, but I wasn't, either. I weighed about 220 pounds at the time, the biggest I had ever been."

The polo shirt incident immediately sparked something inside Annie's father. Standing among the racks of too-small clothes, Annie's dad challenged her to a weight-loss competition. "The only guideline was that we had to do it the healthy way—no diet pills, no starvation!" she says. "Whoever could lose thirty pounds (or come closest) by the following October

> *A Healthy Tipping Point is a journey with no final destination.*

would win." After declaring weight-loss war in the middle of the store, Annie and her father started off on an incredible journey.

From that day forward, Annie made a promise to herself. "I would do something active every day, cut my portion sizes, and journal my food intake," she says. "For the rest of the school year and the entire summer, I promised myself that I would do an average of one hour of physical activity a day. I would bike, swim, walk, or garden."

Sticking to her healthy eating and exercise program made Annie more confident in her athletic abilities, and she decided to try out for her school's volleyball team. As part of tryouts, Annie was required to attend pre-season practice for four hours a day for two weeks. "It was like nothing I had ever done before," she admits, recalling the difficult drills. "But it made me realize that I could do anything."

Not only did Annie score a spot on the volleyball team, but she continued to lose weight and get stronger. When it came time to check in with her father about their weight-loss challenge, Annie was proud to report she had lost twenty-two pounds in six months—the healthy way. Her father had lost fifteen pounds. "At first, I never believed it would be possible for us to lose this much weight by just eating right and exercising, but it is amazing what you can accomplish when you put your mind to it. I actually feel healthier, too!" Annie says happily. "My whole family, as well as my doctor, is very proud of me."

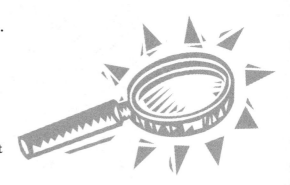

The weight-loss competition with her dad pushed Annie closer to her Healthy Tipping Point. Sociologists coined the term "tipping point" to refer to the moment when a previously unknown or unaccepted phenomenon suddenly becomes widely recognized and accepted. A Healthy Tipping Point is an "aha!" moment when an individual finally realizes that there is no quick-fix solution to health. It's when we no longer exercise just because we're *expected* to and begin to lead active lives because we actually *want* to. When the Healthy Tipping Point occurs, we stop the obsession with thinness and begin to pursue our own Healthy Ideal. It's the moment when we stop saying, "I'll be happy when I lose twenty pounds," or "Maybe I'll go on that vacation when I finally look good in a bikini."

A Healthy Tipping Point is a journey with no final destination. It's about healthy living *for life*, not for looks.

Like Annie, Beth used healthy methods to lose twenty pounds while she was in college, but she didn't experience her true Healthy Tipping Point for several more years. "To be honest, my fitness journey had always been motivated by vanity," Beth, now thirty years old and living in San Francisco, admits. "For the last nine years, I've been working toward smaller hips, buffer arms, a flatter tummy, and a tighter butt. I want to go down a size. I appreciate the fact that good health comes from all this hard work. But truthfully, if you were to ask me why I take such good care of myself, my first response would likely be, 'Because I'd be fat if I didn't!'"

But everything changed for Beth when her close

friend fell ill with pulmonary hypertension. "In the span of a month, an otherwise healthy thirty-one-year-old woman went from living her life normally to being scheduled for an emergency heart and double lung transplant," Beth says. "Visiting her in the hospital made me scared, sad, and anxious." It also forced Beth to reevaluate her own attitude toward health and wellness.

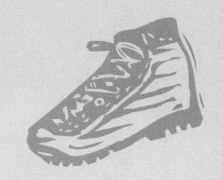

Watching her friend struggle through her operations was "my real Healthy Tipping Point," she says. "Being fit and healthy is not a given. It's a gift. Instead of running one more mile to burn one hundred extra calories, I should run that mile because my heart and my lungs allow me to do so—because my body is privileged and powerful enough to do so." Instead of focusing on her short-term goals, Beth says she is "choosing to focus on the full scope of my fitness accomplishments and how they contribute to my pretty amazing life. My body may have a few wrinkles, dimples, rolls, and folds, but it's also carried me through three half marathons, countless hikes, and treks across some of the most amazing cities in the world. That's something to appreciate and be thankful for every day."

Beth • 30 • San Francisco, California

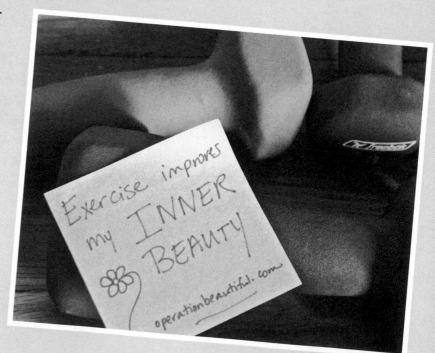

Exercise improves my INNER BEAUTY
operationbeautiful.com

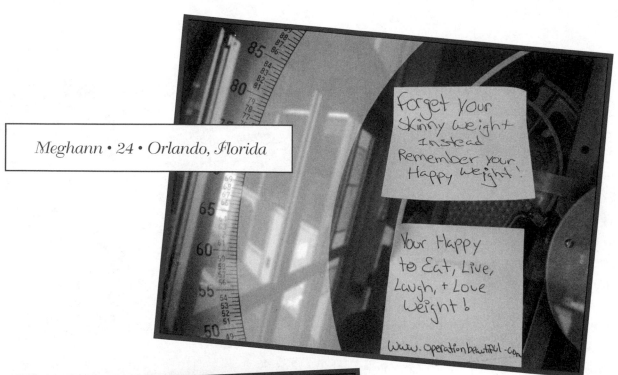

"I used chalk to write this Operation Beautiful note while on a run. It was right beside a bus stop, and I hope lots of people saw it!"

"After my older son was born in 2000, I lost fifty pounds on diet pills. After meeting my husband and getting 'comfortable,' I gained forty or fifty pounds back. I was diagnosed with multiple sclerosis in January 2009, and I was in so much pain that I quit exercising. Coupled with my new medication, I gained another forty more pounds in about six months' time. Today, I'm on new medicine that has helped tremendously—I have very little pain and much more energy. I'm excited

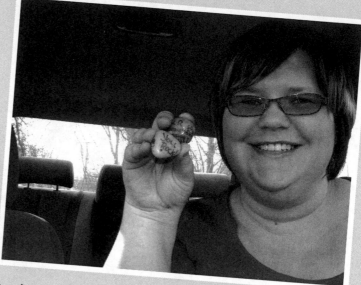

to be active again and lose some weight. But in the meantime, Operation Beautiful has reminded me that we, as women, are beautiful beings. We have the ability to grow a life inside us. Sometimes it takes trials to remind us how strong we are. But I know that a disease or a number on a scale does not define who I am. I am an amazing and beautiful woman. With that thought in mind, I went on a little Operation Beautiful adventure. I had some of those craft rocks that you can use to fill vases so I used a marker to write messages all over them. During my lunch hour, I went to our local park and dropped them along the walking path."

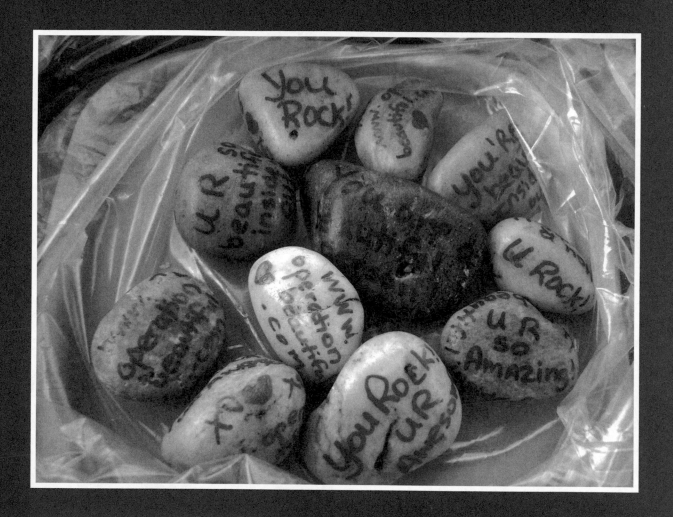

Jamie Habermaas • 31 •
Wayne City, Illinois

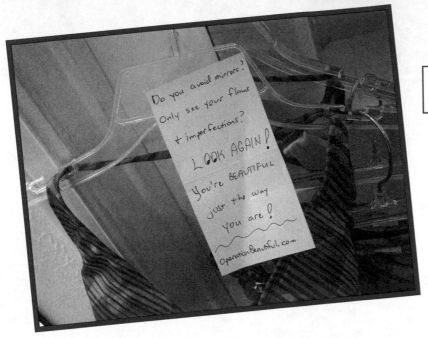

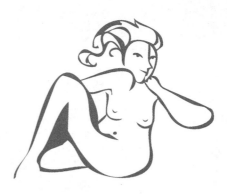

Jana • 46 • Garland, Texas

"*The women's locker room at a gym can often be an intimidating place. I was always one to hide behind the curtain of the private changing rooms. Operation Beautiful has helped me embrace the fact that women come in all shapes and sizes. I no longer hide behind that curtain, and it's the most liberating feeling in the world. I know that I am beautiful inside and out. I thought the women at my gym could be reminded of their beauty.*"

Amy M. • 28 • Ottawa. Ontario, Canada

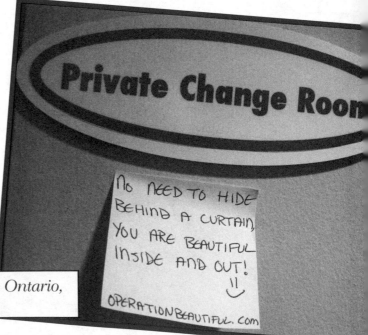

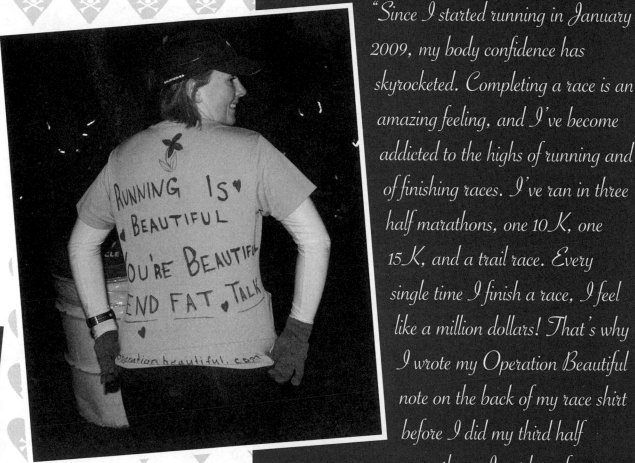

Amber Y. • 21 • Kamloops, British Columbia, Canada

"Since I started running in January 2009, my body confidence has skyrocketed. Completing a race is an amazing feeling, and I've become addicted to the highs of running and of finishing races. I've ran in three half marathons, one 10 K, one 15 K, and a trail race. Every single time I finish a race, I feel like a million dollars! That's why I wrote my Operation Beautiful note on the back of my race shirt before I did my third half marathon. I got lots of compliments on the shirt throughout the race, and I hope that the message touched other people who were running and lifted them up when they felt tired and down!"

"I have been overweight all my life. It's been a constant physical and emotional struggle. I know that I can get to my goal weight one day, but more importantly, I have come to terms with this is who I am. Whether I am 195 or 155 pounds, the thing that matters is that I feel healthy and beautiful. I have always wanted to run a marathon, and I am going to wear this note on my bib number for every upcoming race as I train to reach that goal."

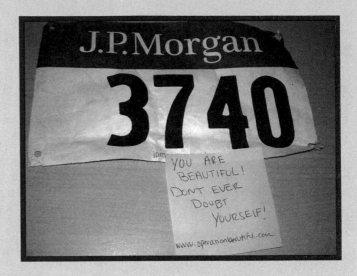

Ashley Niven • 24 • Boston, Massachusetts

"A little more than a year ago, I was overweight and too embarrassed to go to the gym. I was 5'1", 189 pounds, and incredibly depressed. I did not know anything about losing weight in a healthy way, and I always felt like I had to go to the gym to lose weight. I went a few times, but I felt so self-conscious because I was surrounded by people in great shape. That's when I decided to try running outside. It took me about six minutes to run a quarter of a mile, and that was all I could do. It took me about three weeks to work up to running one mile, and I think I cried. I was so

Adriana G. • 23 • California

relieved to find an exercise where I could just zone out and not dread being judged. I adjusted my diet and more than a year later, I have lost sixty-four pounds! I am also in pre-training for the Los Angeles Marathon."

Be Proud! You did something today to nourish your mind, body, and soul! Way to go!

www.operationbeautiful.com

Kristin J. • 29 • La Crosse, Wisconsin

"About ten years ago, I weighed almost two hundred pounds and was an unhealthy, inactive college student. For some reason, my mom and I decided to train and do a triathlon together. I joined the YMCA, and the spinning instructor invited me to one of her classes. She told me that it would be challenging, but to keep trying and eventually it would get easier. Now, I teach spinning, Zumba, and Group Strength classes! I love it because I can give back to people what that one instructor gave to me. Today, I got to my spin class early and taped these notes on every bike. I told my participants to take one home, leave it there, or pass it on. It felt great! I even left a special note for the instructor who would teach after me."

"As a two-time cancer survivor training for my second marathon, I must say that Operation Beautiful has truly changed my life. I get down sometimes about how my hair is thinner, even though it has grown back, or how the tumors in my brain caused me to gain weight. When I remind others about inner beauty, it makes me see and feel my own. I always keep spare notes and sketches in my bag! Keep sharing the love; it's incredible what a few kind words can do for someone."

Hannah Tropicana • 17 • Boston, Massachusetts

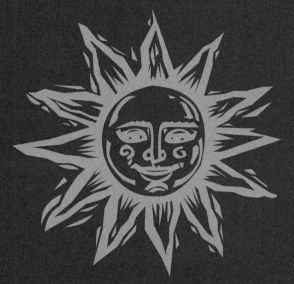

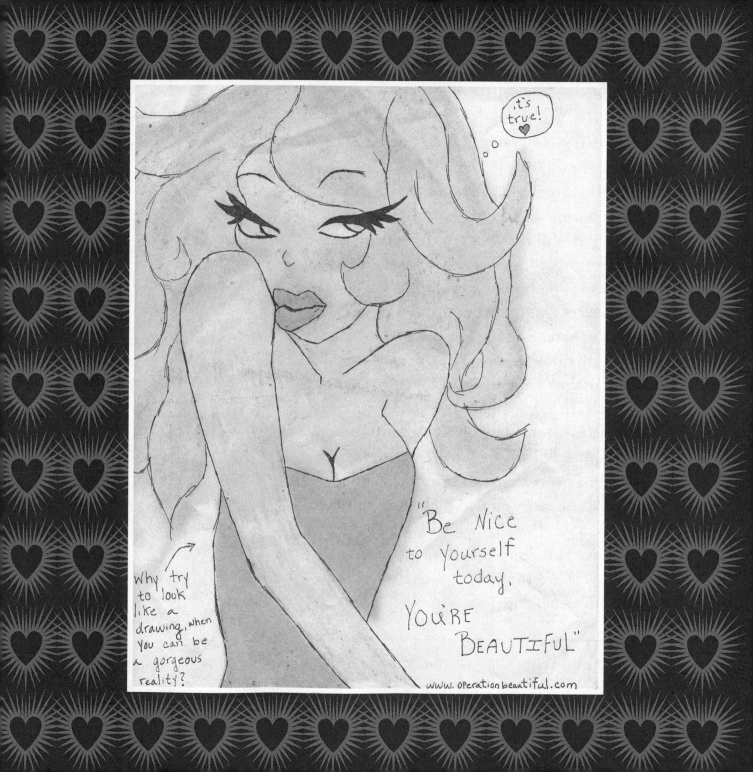

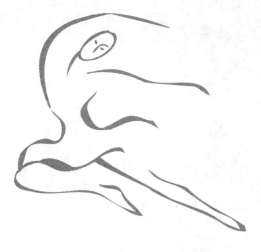

"I'm no longer the girl I was 225 pounds and two years ago, but even when I shed the weight, a part of that girl stayed with me. She is the one who I see when I look in the mirror. That's the girl who was too afraid to go to the gym during peak hours until she'd lost about sixty pounds. She's the girl who hasn't taken the spinning class she's wanted to take for two years. She's the girl who sometimes hates leaving the house just to go to the store, never mind the gym, because she hates her body so intensely she can't imagine how others can look at her with anything other than disdain. I lost the weight, but the self-consciousness never left. I'm working through my body image issues through 'Baby Steps to Body Love Challenge,' in which I step out of my comfort zone and challenge myself to do something that makes me a little uncomfortable. I've challenged myself to go to a yoga class. This seems to work for me—it's really, really hard sometimes, but I rarely back down from a challenge!"

Jenny Weiss • 25 • Boston, Massachusetts

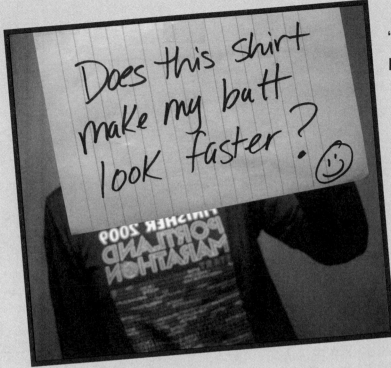

Sherri Becker • 49 • Seattle, Washington

"I saw this phrase on shirts at the Portland Marathon Expo and was inspired to write it on an Operation Beautiful note and leave it on the mirror in the ladies' lounge of our hotel. Come marathon morning, you could hear women laughing and sharing the phrase with each other as they came out of the lounge. Someone pulled out a marker and the next thing you knew, a dozen new friends were writing the saying on the back of their running shirts! We are all shapes and sizes. We are strong, and we are athletes. We are beautiful!"

"I was diagnosed with social anxiety disorder (agoraphobia) when I was fifteen years old. People with agoraphobia will panic in big, crowded areas. School, malls, concerts, and even gyms would throw me into an anxiety attack. I would hyperventilate, sweat, shake, and even vomit. When I started panicking, I honest to goodness felt like my life was in danger and would have to get out of my environment immediately.

I was chubby as a teen and it extended into university. I always wanted to lose the weight and get fit. But the idea of entering a big gym full of strangers would throw me into a panic. Instead, I worked out in my living room or at the pool where I could hide in the water. But as I dropped the weight, I got more energetic and wanted to add more to my workout routine. I started with twenty minutes a week at the campus gym. A year and a half later, I am a triathlete who belongs to one of those big swanky gyms. I'm there almost every day in workout clothes, sweating alongside dozens of people I've never met.

The big change for me came when something my psychologist told me finally clicked—other people really aren't looking at me. Most people are too self-absorbed to notice other strangers in the room, especially at the gym, where we're all distracted by our iPods, weight sets, and cardio intervals. Most importantly, I realized the people at the gym are no different than me. We all started somewhere and deal with many of the same insecurities. People at the gym aren't judging me. If anything we share a common goal—to be as healthy and fit as we can be, no matter where we are on that journey."

Susan Ehrhardt • 23 • Moncton, New Brunswick, Canada

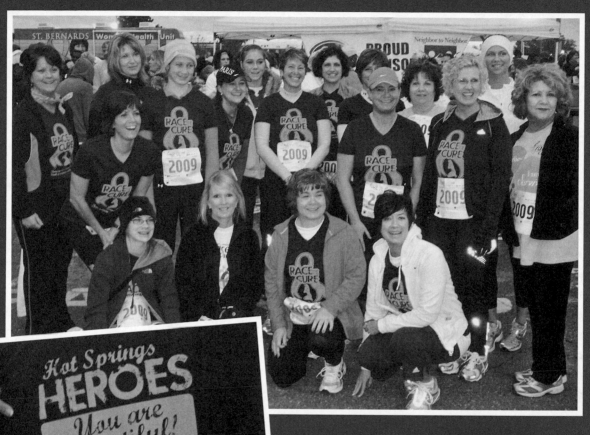

"Last year, I did my first 5K at the Race for the Cure here in Arkansas. This year I am doing it again, but fifty pounds lighter!"

Lorrie • 40 • Hot Springs, Arkansas

THE EXERCISE HABIT

Whether you're a former fitness junkie who fell off the wagon or someone who's never stepped inside a gym, developing a taste for exercise is easier than you think.

- Consider what's holding you back. People avoid exercising because they believe it's too hard or they don't think they have the time. In actuality, a healthier lifestyle is the sum of many small decisions and efforts. To get started, try going for a fast-paced walk around the block or taking your dusty bicycle out of the garage for a spin. Instead of spending your evenings zoning out in front of the television, dance around your living room for a fun cardio workout. Remember that even the healthiest woman you know started from scratch.

- You can cultivate the inner drive to get out there and sweat. Track your progress by keeping a workout diary, make a list of the reasons why you want to get healthy, or join an online support group or message board. Tell your friends and family about your plan to get healthy and ask them to check in on you from time to time.

- Create a plan of action. To prepare your plan, enlist the help of a friend who is knowledgeable

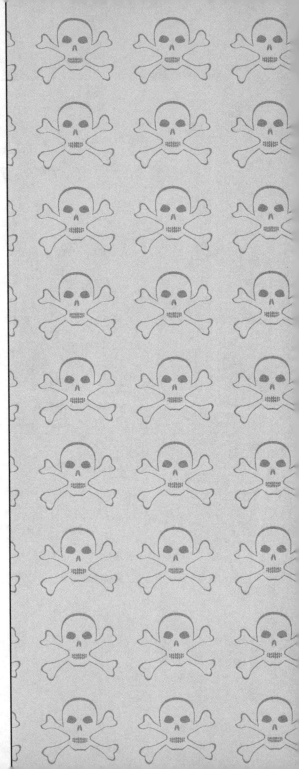

about healthy exercise, your doctor, or a personal trainer. Describe your goals, which should be quantifiable and might include losing a certain number of pounds, reducing your blood pressure, being able to do ten push-ups, or running a 5K race. Your goals should include one or two large goals, as well as many smaller, more easily attainable "milestone goals." Identifying milestone goals will reinforce your behavior and help keep you on track. Next, write down the steps necessary to achieve these goals so you have a clear under-standing of your new path. Last, recognize that it may take weeks or even months to accomplish your goals. Be patient—it's worth it!

· Positively reinforce your behavior. Prepare a list of rewards for each goal you achieve, as it will give you something to look forward to and work toward. It's most effective if your goals are not food-related, as tying reward/punishment to eating is a slippery slope. Examples of great rewards include a back massage, manicure, new pair of pants, or a nice, long bubble bath. The "value" of your rewards should increase as you move toward your larger, more general goals.

· Work interval training to your advantage! Interval training consists of periods of high-intensity exercises followed by a period of recovery exercises. These "sprints" are repeated. You can do interval training on any cardio machine or while running, swimming, bicycling, or even dancing! Repeating two minutes of high intensity exercise with one minute of recovery exercise (for example) helps beat workout boredom, revs your metabolism, and can be more effective than just chugging along at a moderate pace. Run/walk intervals are also a great way to progress from walking or jogging to running.

- Stop punishing yourself. So many women try to guilt, bribe, or trick themselves into exercising, but punishment simply does not create a lifelong love of working out. All you're doing is training yourself to hate exercise.

- Don't set yourself up to fail. Failure can be very disheartening, so it's important to set achievable goals. For example, don't take a solemn vow to work out five days a week when you know it will be difficult to exercise more than three times. Do the best you can at any given point in time. Your best is subject to many external factors, such as your work schedule or general fitness level.

- Find a workout buddy to inspire and motivate you. Working out with someone else also makes it more fun! Caroline's buddy was someone she already knew. "Running randomly came up in the conversation, and she wanted to join in," says Caroline, a

twenty-four-year-old from Athens, Georgia. "We both know how much someone holding you accountable helps get you off the couch." Mica found a workout buddy in a more unexpected way—on the Internet! "I put an ad for a running partner on the Strictly Platonic section of Craigslist," says Mica, a twenty-three-year-old from Champaign, Illinois. "Knowing that she is waiting with laced running shoes has gotten me out the door on some of the windiest, rainiest, and coldest days imaginable."

· Anticipate challenges to your workout routine, such as during the holidays or stressful times in your personal life. Be aware of when you'll be tempted to slack off, and take proactive steps to ensure you stick with your healthy habits. Pack your gym bag the night before or arrange to meet up with your workout buddy in the morning.

· Instead of shying away from new physical activities, relish your inexperience! Sign up for a salsa class or try indoor rock climbing. You'll never know what you like—or are surprisingly good at—unless you try. "I was overweight my entire life until a defining moment made me realize I needed to make a change," says Emily J., a twenty-three-year-old from Toronto. "I still get nervous when trying something new. It took me months to finally start going to yoga, and without the firm push of a friend, I'm not sure I would have. But the positive atmosphere of a yoga class is what appeals to me more than the practice itself: It is such a supportive, uplifting community!"

- Exercise for the right reasons. Regular exercise reduces your risk of diseases such as cancer and heart disease, decreases stress, boosts your mood, and helps you sleep better. You're more likely to stick with an exercise program if you're focused on the long-term benefits than just simply having washboard abs.

- Get sneaky with your workouts. Exercise does not necessarily equal hours spent slaving away at the gym. Try parking your car farther away from the store entrance, taking the stairs instead of the elevator, playing with your children or pets, or stretching while watching television.

- Cut yourself some slack, and try not to ruminate on skipped workouts—even if you fall off the wagon for a few days, weeks, or even months. "There are always those days when you don't want to work out. You feel like doing nothing, and you aren't motivated. Don't let those days keep you distracted from your goals," says Ashley Spencer, a twenty-three-year-old from Baltimore, Maryland. "Tomorrow is a new day and you can reach your dreams. Your potential is limitless."

Superwoman Syndrome: Past the Breaking Point

One of the hardest things for many women to do is simply say "enough is enough." It seems we are pulled in so many directions by so many different people who are clamoring for our time and attention. Perhaps it's our natural womanly instinct to say, "Yes, of course I will help," or maybe we've just forgotten how to put ourselves first. Regardless of the cause, we often find ourselves overextended and exhausted as we try to be everything to everyone.

The modern woman strives to fulfill a variety of roles, such as employee, student, mother, spouse, friend, volunteer. Life becomes a wild roller-coaster ride from one activity to the next, and at each turn, we're grasping for perfection. Superwoman Syndrome—believing that you can do it all and more—manifests itself most poignantly in our pursuit of the Thin Ideal, especially as it relates to exercise and fitness. As we struggle to keep all of our balls in the air, we're losing track of what should be our utmost priority: our own mental and physical health.

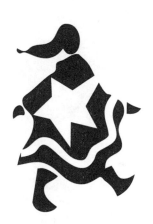

Angela frequently cried herself to sleep and woke up with a headache. She was balancing a stressful job in a field she despised, a two-hour commute, and a rigorous workout schedule that left her feeling burnt out and beat up. "I pushed myself very hard. I was trying to do everything at once," remembers Angela, who is twenty-six years old and lives in Canada. "I used to use exercise as a way to feel in control of my life. Looking back, I had it all wrong, but when someone is in the depths of disordered thinking patterns, it is very hard to recognize that it is actually unhealthy."

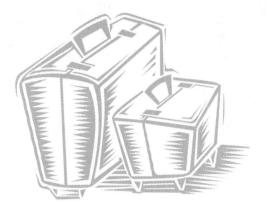

Angela, who has a master's in social psychology, observes that she also fell victim to the Social Comparison Trap, a phenomenon in which a woman constantly compares herself to her close family members and friends, as well as celebrities and models in magazines. "When a woman falls into this trap, there is no longer an internal gauge for success," she notes. "It's a dangerous situation because nothing will ever be good enough. There will always be someone more beautiful, thinner, or more successful." As part of the Social Comparison Trap, women get caught up in a silent competition between each other, striving to 'one-up' the other, even if it's at the expense of their health or sanity.

As Angela watched her friends and family members realize tremendous fitness accomplishments, such as running marathons, she also felt pressured to make her workouts longer and more intense. When she decided to add difficult sprint workouts to her running regime, Angela's body rebelled. She suffered a painful pelvic injury that sidelined her from intense cardio activity for two months.

Angela quickly realized that she wasn't a Superwoman—she was just super overextended.

The time away from the treadmill forced Angela to closely examine why she pushed herself so hard in many areas of her life, including fitness. Acknowledging that she's always been an overachiever, Angela says she now strives to silence her perfectionist tendencies, which often do her more harm than good.

"In the past, I first looked at what other people had achieved, and I based my fitness goals off that. Now, I try to avoid the Superwoman Syndrome by looking internally to create my own personal goals," says Angela. Striving for smaller, realistic fitness milestones that also consider the other factors in her busy schedule have helped Angela find true happiness. She's now healed from her injury and has slowly gotten back into running, completing several half marathons.

"When I decided to ditch the Superwoman Syndrome, I realized that I could still be a 'super' woman, but it would have to be on my own terms," Angela concludes. "I am much happier and more balanced since I have reclaimed my life and focused on what makes me happy, not other people."

"I posted this Operation Beautiful note at Memorial Park in Houston when I went on my ten-mile run this weekend. There is a nice gravel three-mile course that goes around the park, and there must have been over a hundred people out there on Sunday morning! Everyone was there—men and women, kids and teens, people of every shape and form. I know that many runners feel like they need to be fast or skinny to be good runners, but that's not the case! Great runners are appreciative that they can run and have fun doing it!"

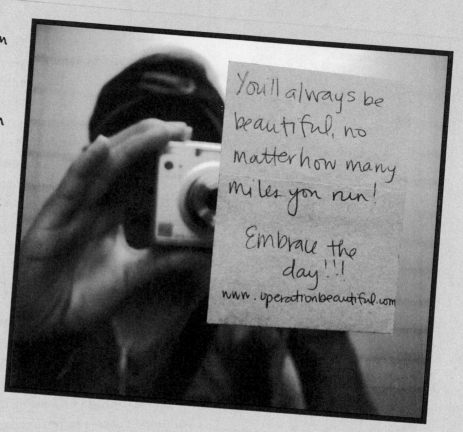

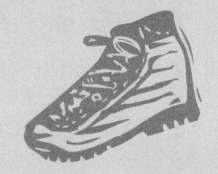

Melissa Schlothan • 24 • California

"I used to be a huge runner, but then got sidelined with a knee injury and had to take multiple months off from intense activity. During this time, it was really hard for me to deal with not being able to run and the slight weight gain that came with it. As with

Taylor Saunders • 22 •
San Luis Obispo, California

any gym locker room, there are mirrors every-where. After I finished a workout and walked to my locker, I would notice myself in the mirror, and negative thoughts would flood my head. After a few days of this, it hit me—what was I thinking? I had just fin-ished working out and doing something great for my body, and all I could do was put myself down! Right away, I wrote myself a little note to stick in my locker that I would see every day, before and after my workout. It reminds me of how strong I am, and how wonderful it is what I'm doing for my body."

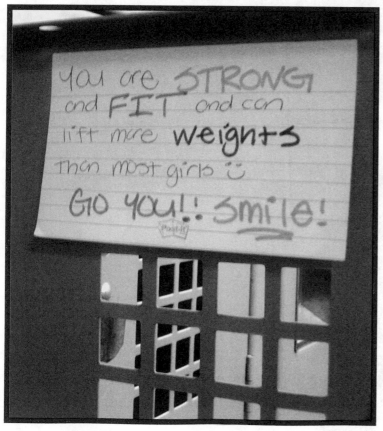

"In March 2009, I was run over by a car while riding my bicycle. The entire right side of my body was run over, including my leg, hip, arm, chest, and my head. Fortunately, I was smart enough to purchase a helmet a few weeks prior and was wearing it the day of my accident. Wearing that helmet saved my life. Your beautiful head deserves to be protected by a helmet."

Kelly A. • 22 • Orlando, Florida

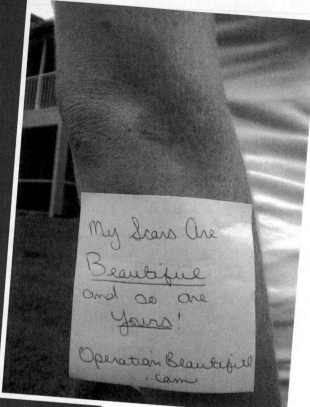

My Scars Are Beautiful and so are Yours! OperationBeautiful.com

"This past weekend, I ran the Tufts Health Plan 10 K for Women in Boston. The race dates back to 1977 and is the largest women's-only 10 K in the nation. I wanted to add to the history of inspiration and empowerment that this race has achieved by showcasing an Operation Beautiful note. I hope my note reminded women that their participation in

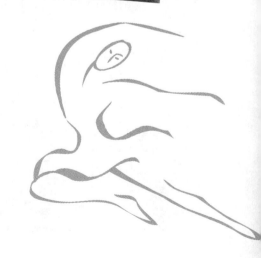

134

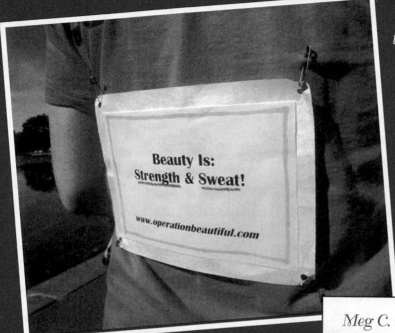

Beauty Is:
Strength & Sweat!

www.operationbeautiful.com

this race is part of what makes them 'beautiful.' Sweat isn't usually thought of as beautiful, but when it's the result of hard work, dedication, and athleticism, nothing could be more beautiful in a woman."

Meg C. • 24 • Boston, Massachusetts

"I try to be Superwoman every single day. Wife, mother, blogger, cook, friend, yoga teacher—all while maintaining my own exercise and personal fitness goals. Yoga has helped me to let go a bit and to try to be more 'roll with it' and less 'control it,' but my innate nature is Type A. It can be hard to always achieve balance, but generally I believe I am successful at it. I think that anytime a person becomes fanatical, dogmatic, or too rigid in eating or in exercise, he or she has usually lost the sense of fun and pleasure that we can derive from these things. I try to keep a lighthearted attitude and choose a little bit of everything, in moderation."

Averie • 33 • Phoenix, Arizona

"All of my friends are thinner than me. It is something that almost always bothers me, even after I lost the twenty-five pounds I had gained in college. One morning a few weeks ago, I did my usual routine of run, shower, and breakfast, but I added in a quick set of push-ups, too. I have been doing a set of push-ups every few days for about six months, and that day I decided to just see how many real push-ups I could do before I got too tired. I did twenty-five push-ups in a row and was shocked and pleased. I'll admit it—I immediately called my husband to tell him how many I did! It doesn't matter that I have a little pudge or that I am a little bigger than my friends, because I am strong. I am beautiful. I was in such a great mood knowing how strong I have become that I decided to share the positive energy—I hope it made someone's day!"

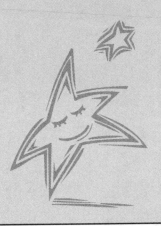

Sabrina Garibian • 26 • Philadelphia, Pennsylvania

WELCOME TO PHILADELPH
YOU ARE IN TAXICAB

YOU ARE BEAUTIFUL
JUST THE WAY YOU ARE.
www.operationbeautiful.com

BE SURE YO
COMMEN

OUR PROPERT
215-683-9440

"Name a body part and I've injured it [from over-exercising]—and injured it badly. At twenty-four years old, I've had multiple stress fractures, a ruptured Achilles tendon, cortisone injections, a broken elbow, and back surgery. I've now literally run myself into rest by fracturing both of my legs (at the same time) this summer. I'm the girl with two medical boots, hobbling around the city and unable to run.

Recently, I was balancing on my two boots during the bus ride to work, grimacing with frustration. Per usual, I received various blank stares and pity-filled pouts from commuters that morning (but no one got up to give me their seat). I did notice one girl staring at me more sincerely, and when she got up to leave the bus, she blindly tossed a Post-it at me. My initial reaction was bitterness and cynicism, but then I looked at the note, which read: 'I hope your legs get better soon. Keep smiling! From: someone who cares.' I smiled a large, true, and natural smile. I looked around and giggled to myself, in utter disbelief that someone actually did that for me. Her five-second gesture took me from sad to oh-so-happy.

Her note made me ponder, 'If a stranger can look at me and deem me worthy, why can't I do the same for myself?' The note helped me realize that I am ready to start living my life. I've ruined running, my one true passion, with notions of 'must do's' and 'have to's', and I'm sick of this dizzying cycle of self-doubt—I'm ready to trust myself. My legs will get better and I will keep smiling. Why me? Why not me?"

Jessica C. • 24 • Boston, Massachusetts

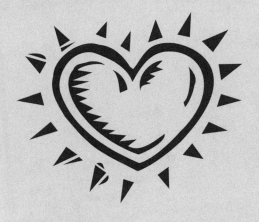

"I am a classic Type A personality and a perfectionist, so I always feel pressured to do everything—to be everything to everybody. Up until twelve weeks ago, I was working out seven days a week—four days of high-impact aerobics classes, three days of regular cardio workouts, and lifting four days a week. I was quickly headed to a burnout and/or serious injury. And then I discovered I was pregnant. Suddenly, I did not have the energy to keep up my training schedule, and my doctor told me that I was doing too much and could put my pregnancy in jeopardy. Now I work out four times a week, under my doctor's supervision. I feel great! I am taking care of my body, which in turn is growing a happy, healthy baby. I am glad that I learned the lesson about balance now, before baby arrives, so that after he/she is here I will have a better understanding of how to balance the needs of my family with my own."

Kimberly L. • 27 • Alma, Georgia

"I work as a dietitian/personal trainer at a local health club, and I decided a good place to put a note was smack-dab in the middle of the scale. During a normal training session, I see about twelve to fifteen people check their weight before a workout. It always amazes me that so many people are so focused on the number on the scale versus the more intrinsic benefits of exercise."

Jessica M. • 25 • Massachusetts

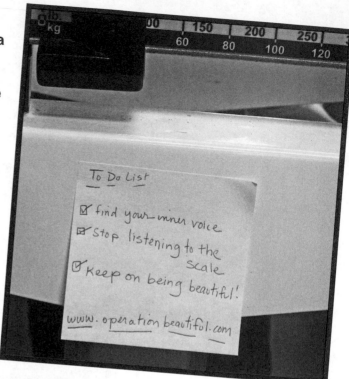

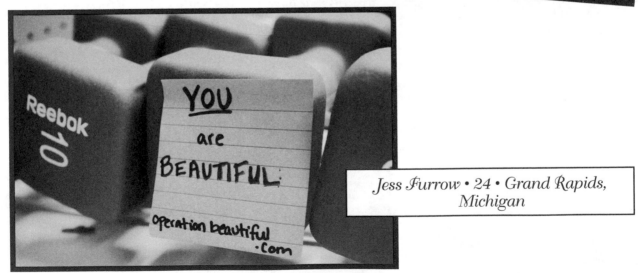

Jess Furrow • 24 • Grand Rapids, Michigan

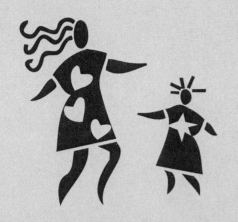

"*I'm a former Fat Talking girl. After fifteen years of feeling sorry for myself and yo-yo dieting, I knew I had to stop the unhealthy cycle for the sake of my newborn son. Four years later, I'm a new woman. Not because I am seventy pounds lighter, but because I stopped focusing on fat. I stopped worrying about what I looked liked in the swimsuit, and I just swam. I stopped shying away from activities. Now I do things instead of thinking about doing them, like running the Baltimore Marathon.*"

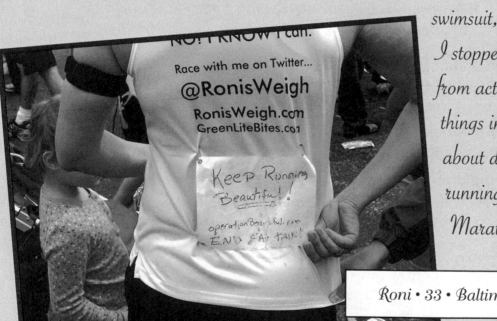

Roni • 33 • Baltimore, Maryland

141

"I grew up surrounded by athletes. I, on the other hand, was a musical theater nerd. I performed in all of the school plays, sang in three of our school's choir groups, and took voice lessons in my spare time. Though I had some of the best friends in the world, I couldn't help but feel inadequate in comparison at times. After I graduated high school and went to college, my confidence plummeted. I found no joy in dressing up and going out on the weekends; I didn't find myself attractive. I felt lazy and unmotivated; I didn't know what to do with all of my newfound free time. I had, once again, found myself becoming friends with girls who had been athletes their whole lives. This only made me feel worse about myself; I definitely referred to myself as the 'f-word' many times during this transition in my life.

There was nothing I wanted more badly than to join a gym and get myself in shape. But I couldn't do it. I was embarrassed. I didn't own athletic sneakers. What would I possibly wear? How long does a person spend at the gym? How do you use the equipment? I was terrified that I would show up and get stared at by people who could see that I didn't belong there. I was afraid I would get laughed at for not knowing how to use an elliptical or the proper way to lift a weight.

It took me five months to swallow my shame and walk into a gym. There were nerves and there was hesitation, but I

did it. And after I went once, I couldn't stop. I was addicted, in a bad way. You see, my intentions from the beginning were never healthy ones. I didn't want to go for the endorphins or the health benefits. I wanted to go because I felt like I should be going. I felt like if everyone else was doing it, I should be doing it as well. Because I hadn't thought to obtain any general knowledge about nutrition, health, or exercise prior to this, I slipped slowly down a path of self-destruction. Exercise turned into over-exercise. It got to the point where I was actually doing sit-ups in the bathroom at work, creating bruises on my back that confused my family and friends. This over-exercise ignited food restriction. As you can imagine, it was a total disaster. In five months, I lost thirty-five pounds, and I didn't even need to lose weight to begin with.

Though it took a long time to grasp the severity of this situation, I did eventually accept recovery and work toward regaining health. Slowly, I began to fit together the pieces of the puzzles that I had overlooked the first time through; primarily proper nutrition and healthy exercise habits. I worked with a nutritionist to create a meal plan, even if it wasn't always easy to follow it. I cut out the gym entirely, taking walks if I ever felt overwhelmingly antsy.

It's been two years, and I am proud to say that all of this is far behind me. Once I reached a healthy weight, I started to go to the gym again. This time, I went for the right reasons. I was no longer embarrassed, and I was no longer afraid. Instead, I was proud of what my body—my healthy body—could do. Now if these negative thoughts try to creep back, I remind myself how strong I am. Not only for what I can do but for what I've overcome and for what I'm capable of doing. I've recently started to train for a half marathon to prove to myself that I am good enough, despite what I've tried to convince myself in the past.

I've wasted too much time being afraid of the unknown, and I refuse to live my life like that anymore."

Alyssa • 21 • New Jersey

"I left this note on the scale at the gym I go to. I saw women agonizing over two pounds up or down every time I went there, and it pained me. I spent years trapped inside an eating disorder, and actually have spent the past year and a half recovering from the relapse that nearly killed me. No one thought I would make it without the aid of a medical team and a treatment facility. But I did. I recovered on my own. I am alive, and I am finally beginning to realize that it doesn't matter what I weigh—I am always going to be the same person inside, and that is who I need to love. And so I posted that note there because I felt other people needed to be

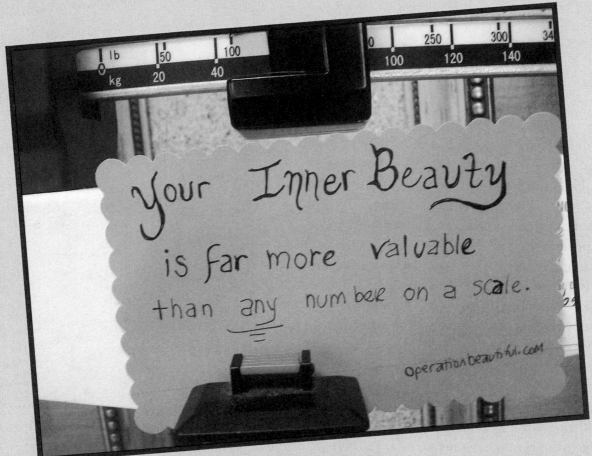

told that as well. I figured it would be taken down by the next time I went for my strength-training session, but it was still there on the scale! That note was left there for about two weeks, and I even caught a few smiles born as people saw what it said."

Tori • 21 • Stratford, Connecticut

Emotional Exercise

Exercise produces feel-good endorphins, which flood the brain to boost our confidence and mood. However, just as pursuing the unattainable Thin Ideal can produce negative emotions, our fitness habits can be destructive if we do not approach our workouts in a healthy, balanced manner.

When they miss a workout, some women may feel guilty, throw their hands up in disgust, and think, "Well, I've done it now—I might as well eat this entire pint of ice cream for dinner." Other women might react to a skipped workout by overcompensating the next day, pushing too hard and risking injury. For others, the gym may produce feelings of inferiority ("Why aren't I as fast/thin/strong as that person?") or anxiety ("Everyone is watching me screw up this yoga pose!").

Here are some simple steps for taking the negativity out of your workout:

- It's important that we use exercise as a positive outlet for our energy and stress, not a punishment. Feelings of stress, guilt, anxiety, and dread are not normal reactions to a less-than-stellar workout. Acknowledging unhealthy reactions to exercise is

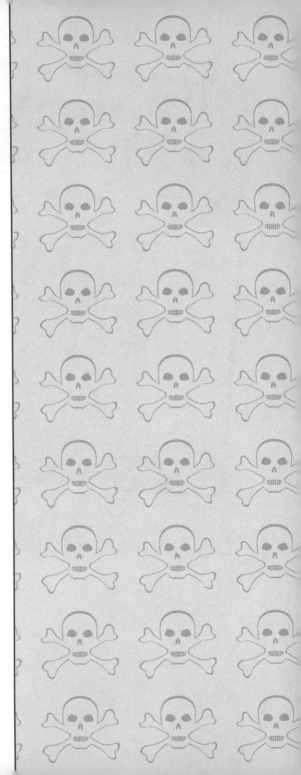

very important for your physical, as well as mental, health. After all, it's hard to make something a lifelong habit if you secretly resent it.

- Recognize that negative reactions to exercise are part of the larger Superwoman Syndrome—the belief that we must be able to do it all (and do it perfectly to boot). If you struggle with feelings of inadequacy, give yourself permission to not be perfect. This simple act can be very powerful and freeing.

- Ditch the All-or-Nothing attitude and adopt the Something-Is-Better-Than-Nothing approach. "Moderation is very important in the journey to health," says Beth Phillips, a twenty-four-year-old from Washington, D.C., who struggled with the Superwoman Syndrome in the past. If the day is particularly busy, and you cannot squeeze in a full-length workout, do sit-ups while watching television or squats while cooking dinner. When you just feel too lazy or too tired, allow yourself to zone out with a book or swap your sweaty workouts with a casual stroll after dinner. "I now realize that I only have this one body for the rest of my whole life, so I have to be kind to it," says Beth.

- Take the macro approach to assessing your healthy lifestyle. We've been trained to think about our fitness (and eating) habits in terms of twenty-four-hour blocks when, in actuality, our bodies don't have an internal clock that resets at the stroke of midnight! Thinking about your health in terms of weekly blocks is more positive, reaffirming, and realistic. Instead of saying, "I skipped my workout today," remind yourself that you already worked out two times this week, which is an accomplishment.

- Avoid the Social Comparison Trap by setting goals that reflect your current fitness level and abilities. Instead of trying to one-up other women, look toward balanced, healthy role models for motivation to be the best you can be.

- Remember that your mental health is just as important—if not more so—than your physical fitness. Meditation can be an invigorating way to begin your day or a calming way to fall asleep. To ease yourself into a quiet state of mind, turn the lights down and sit cross-legged or lie flat on your back. Close your eyes, and focus on the sound and feeling of your breathing. To help yourself relax, visualize a safe or happy place from your memory. Alternatively, try Positive Thinking Meditation, in which you imagine yourself accomplishing your goals for the day. Use phrases like, "I will be able to do . . ." and "I will easily finish . . ." Above all, don't be afraid to sit in silence! If your mind wanders (which is normal), just gently bring it back to a quiet state.

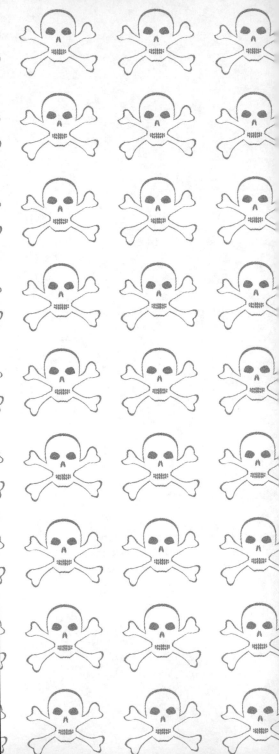

- Listen to your body's cues. Injuries (such as a strained ligament or a stress fracture) and mental burn-out are the most obvious signs that you are overdoing it on exercise. When your body reacts negatively to exercise, it is highly likely that you have been ignoring or burying the emotional cues that enough is enough.

Chapter 5

Food

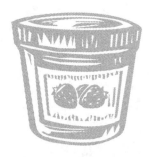

Perhaps the most ironic—and troubling—part of our obsession with the Thin Ideal is that most women are, in fact, medically overweight. In fact, nearly one-third of American adults are overweight, and another third are obese. The difference between what we *want* to look like and what we *actually* look like grows—literally—every year. Confronted with expanding waistlines, more than two-thirds of adult women say they're trying to lose weight at any given time. Americans spend more than $46 billion on diet pills, shakes, bars, books, and strange contraptions that promise to whittle your middle into an appealing six-pack.

Are your pants a little tight? Are you unhappy with your looks? Are you yearning to fit into that bathing suit before your big vacation? Don't worry—with a diet, you'll have *amazing* results in just a few days. All you

> *If our diets aren't working, why are we so obsessed with them?*

have to do is eat a low-carb diet; shun all forms of fat; consume lots of protein; dine like you live near the Mediterranean Sea; avoid white-colored foods; don't eat past 8:00 P.M.; plan your meals in a certain carbohydrate to protein to fat ratio; or just forgo real, solid food entirely and drink a milk shake instead. You may be miserable for a few weeks, but any diet book worth its metaphorical weight will tell you that the deprivation, hunger, and annoyance is worth it . . . *right*?

Wrong. Much of the time, money, and energy we spend on diets is entirely wasted. More than half of dieters regain the weight they lose within a year, and nearly all dieters regain the weight in five years. Research has found that yo-yo dieting is harmful to our immune systems and metabolism. Most diets simply don't produce real, long-lasting, and maintainable results. If our diets aren't working, why are we so obsessed with them?

For so many of us, diets represent everything we are lacking in our normal lifestyles. Many women—and men—feel out of control with their everyday style of eating. Most people do not eat with a sense of purpose; they just eat whatever food is available, fast, and cheap. Diets provide us with structure, and a clear understanding of what we need to do to be "healthy." Yet more than anything else, dieting gives us hope—hope that we one day may fit that Thin Ideal.

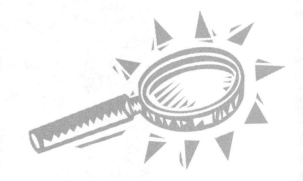

Somewhere along the way, we became convinced

that dieting would make us thin, and thinness would make us happy.

Katie McLaughlin, a twenty-four-year-old, was a self-confessed yo-yo dieter. "I spent years eating in cycles or phases: restrict, binge, repeat," says Katie. "There was no balance for me; either I was avoiding food at all costs or eating everything in sight." Like many dieters, Katie found it impossible to stick to her meal plan, which consisted of eating mostly frozen portion-controlled dinners. "I rarely lasted more than a month on a diet. I would restrict my food intake so much that after four weeks of feeling hungry and deprived, my body would completely revolt and I would end up bingeing on everything in sight," she admits. "Any weight that I had lost in those four weeks returned in half the time, plus more."

When she was a college sophomore, Katie carried around a swimsuit catalog as a reminder to stick to her diet. She had a beach vacation planned with a friend and her friend's family, and Katie was determined to feel comfortable—and look good—in her bathing suit. "I thought that looking at the models and their stereotypically ideal bodies would be motivation for me to continue moderating my food intake like a hawk. I carried that catalog with me everywhere. If I was feeling the urge to veer off my diet, I'd pull it out and remind myself that summer was just around the corner," remembers Katie. When Katie finally did find a bathing suit that fit her well and made her feel comfortable, she snatched it up. "It was magical. I don't know what it was about that bathing suit. It was nothing special—just a plain black one-piece with a halter neck. But it slimmed me in all the right places, and I was thrilled."

Katie ditched the swimsuit catalog. Instead, she hung her new bathing suit on the back of her bedroom door. It was only February, many months until her vacation, so Katie continued to diet in anticipation of wearing her new bathing suit. After a few weeks of perfect eating, she would reach a breaking point, overeat, and skip her workouts for several days. When she rebelled against her strict, self-imposed diet, Katie would feel guilty and restrict her intake again, restarting the vicious cycle. "I completely lost touch with my body—particularly my hunger and fullness cues—because I didn't trust my body to tell me what it needed," she says. "Instead I trusted magazines, commercials, and advertisements to tell me what to eat and not to eat. I looked to society to tell me I looked good, instead of looking to my body to tell me it felt good."

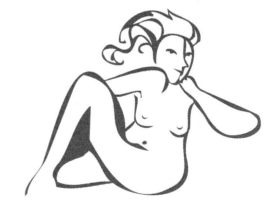

The vacation at the beach ended up being a real wake-up call for Katie. Her beloved bathing suit caught on a lounge chair and ripped the very first day. "To say I was horrified would be an extreme understatement," says Katie. In hindsight, she believes that her passion for the perfect bathing suit and patterns of dieting were symptomatic of an issue

Katie McLaughlin • 24 •
Baltimore, Maryland

Look **10** lbs Lighter in **10** seconds®

You don't need a miracle... you're already beautiful!

operationbeautiful.com

Miraclesuit®

much more complex than how much she weighed. "My fixation with the scale was merely masking heavier feelings of inadequacy," she admits. "At the time I couldn't peel away the layers and see what was really missing in my life, things like balance and forgiveness and relaxation. That little hole in my swimsuit represented a much bigger hole in my life. As that black thread unraveled, so did my supposed self-confidence. I wasn't truly living my life; it was being lived without me, while I remained buried in a weight-loss magazine or a swimsuit catalog."

Katie's revelation that dieting was not only holding her back mentally but was also ineffective for losing and maintaining weight was life-altering. "Turns out that when I stopped obsessing about food, weight, and dieting, I had a lot of extra time, which I used to explore new hobbies like yoga and healthy cooking," Katie says. "In the end, I learned that my true beauty—and everyone's, for that matter—is not static. Our true beauty emerges and grows out of the process of turning inward and learning to appreciate what we find there. By taking the time to explore what makes us beautiful and special and valuable, we actually become even more beautiful than we were before."

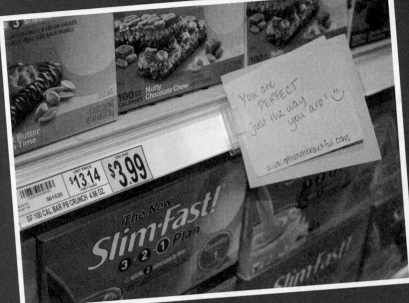

Alyssa • 21 • Los Angeles, California

"At my grocery store, all of the diet products are kept in the same aisle as toiletries. This means that if I want to buy shampoo or conditioner, I have to face shelves upon shelves of 'metabolism boosters' and Slim-Fast cans. There is nothing worse than passing a young girl standing before these products, stocking up on the latest diet quick fix. Thinking of society's skewed perceptions of beauty has always weighed heavy on my heart. I've wasted enough time and energy picking myself apart in the mirror, and I absolutely hate thinking of all the other people going through the same thing. Even if only one person sees my note, then it is good enough for me. It may not make a difference in the world, but I truly hope that it made some girl feel beautiful, even if it was only for a second."

"A few years ago, I decided to take control of my poor eating habits and join Weight Watchers. While a member of Weight Watchers, I was always looking for support. I really needed someone to tell me that I was okay the way I was. I posted this note in a <u>Weight Watchers</u> magazine because I know there were others just like me looking for comfort and nice words. I am hoping that the person who finds this knows they are perfect and beautiful the way they are!"

Kristi • 24 • Milwaukee, Wisconsin

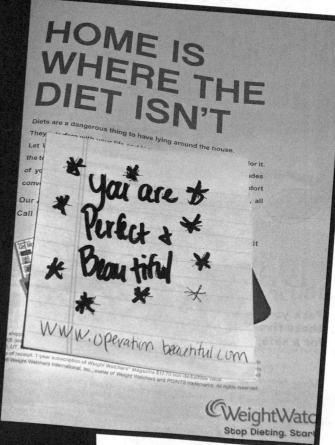

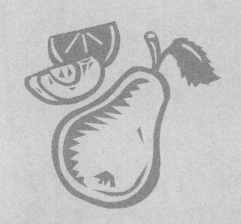

"I've yo-yoed back and forth between overweight and obese since college. I've tried almost every diet in the book. Two years ago, I tipped the scales at 230 pounds. For my 5' 4" frame, that was just too much, and I had constant joint and back problems. Every time I tried a new weight-loss plan, I'd drop ten pounds quickly, revel in my 'success' by eating all the junk I had deprived myself of, and then beat myself up emotionally for 'blowing it.' Before I knew it, I had gained back the weight, and then some.

Now I realize that this journey cannot be about weight loss. If all I care about is not being fat, then I'm setting myself up to fail, because I am sending a message to my soul that I am not acceptable, not worthy, not beautiful, unless I can shed the pounds. If I can't love myself now, will that really change just because I drop a dress size or two?

My mom once told me she didn't understand how I could be so intelligent, so successful, so organized about everything besides my own health. That was a wake-up call, because she didn't refer to it as my weight—she referred to it as my health. And that's really what this is about. Seeking a more active, healthy lifestyle that gives me the energy I need to do all the things I love—making my twelve-hour shifts as a nurse a little more bearable for my feet; going on adventures with my partner, Steve; getting my body into shape so that I can give birth to healthy children and be able to chase after them; and reducing my risk for chronic disease so that I can grow old and thrive and see my children have children, and their children have children!

Above all else, it's about looking in the mirror TODAY and seeing a beautiful woman. If that is the message my soul receives, then every day is a victory and there are no failures."

Kristine H. • 29 • Portland, Oregon

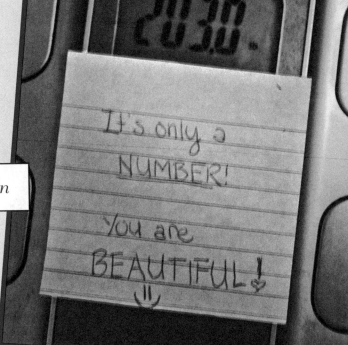

162

"When my digestive illness began, I had no idea what was going on with my body. Because of the constant, massive bloating I was experiencing, I incorrectly assumed that I got fat. My medical diagnosis of colonic inertia explained my bloating, but the disordered thoughts and actions that came with it did not go away. As a result of thinking I was fat, I had fallen into patterns of restrictive eating, bingeing, attempts at purging, and, once I learned how to control the bloating, compulsive exercise.

The compulsive exercising had taken a toll on my knees, and the doctor ordered rest. I dreaded all the weight I was going to gain without exercise. At the same time, I had started to read about the benefits of real, whole foods and began eating cleanly—for the first time, I avoided anything labeled 'low carb' or 'fat free.' After a few months of barely exercising, I was surprised to find that I felt and looked better than ever. As I started slowly incorporating exercise back into my life, I realized that all the negative thoughts that pushed me to over-exercise were gone. I was working out when I wanted for the amount of time I wanted. For the first time in a long time, I was treating my body with respect. As a result, my entire thought process changed and my disordered thoughts and behaviors faded.

Although I still suffer from digestive problems and extreme bloating, I know now that all the time I spent letting negative thoughts about my body consume me was futile. My life became a vicious cycle of negative thoughts and unhealthy actions. Once I treated my body with love, these negative thoughts subsided. Bloat or no bloat, fat or no fat, I am beautiful. And so are you."

Dori Manela • 26 • New York

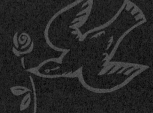

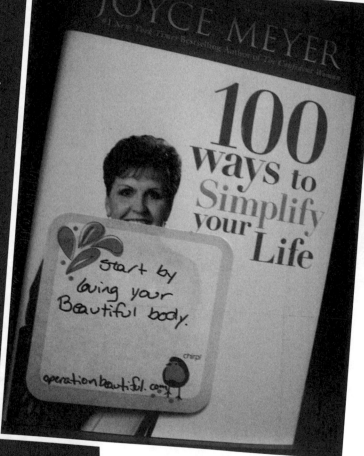

Heather O'Donnell • 31 •
Colby, Wisconsin

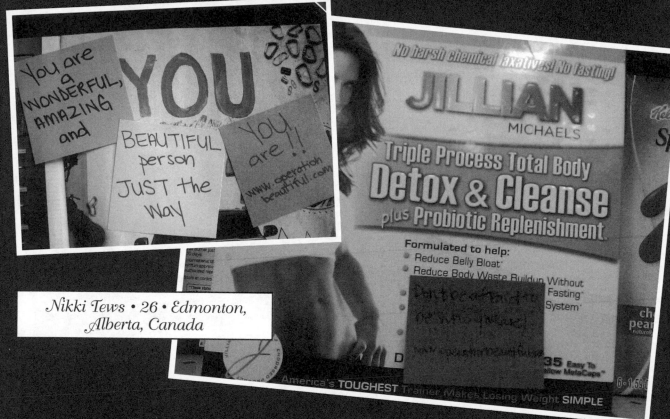

Nikki Tews • 26 • Edmonton,
Alberta, Canada

"I posted this note at a diet clinic, which I get frustrated with because any diet that cuts out healthy fats or fruit doesn't seem like it's healthy at all! I have never believed in 'diets.' I try my best to stay healthy by eating right and doing regular exercise. I'm by no means skinny (I would call myself average), but I'm happy and I feel generally healthy and good about myself."

Melissa Schlothan • 24 •
California

"For as long as I can remember, I have struggled with self-esteem and confidence, so much so that I've missed out on jobs, new friendships, and other opportunities. I turned thirty-one years old this year and promised myself that my thirties were not going to be like my teens and twenties. I do not need anyone else's validation. When I do my errands, I fill the Main Street with little pink Post-it notes! My favorite place to put them is on racks of clothes, in changing rooms, and in magazines. I love to choose magazines directed at dieters or young women, open a random page, and stick on my little piece of inspiration. I can't even put into words how much this simple act of kindness has boosted my self-esteem, my confidence, and my love for life."

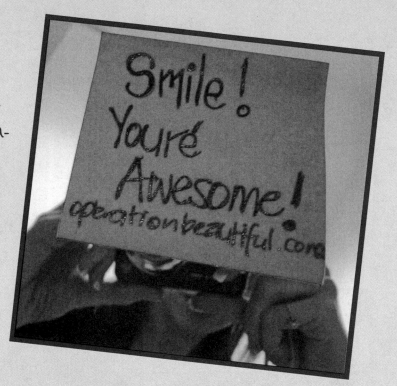

Jandy Resch-Pitts • 31 •
Melbourne, Victoria, Australia

"This is the first Operation Beautiful note I posted. I put it up in the dessert section of a French supermarket I go to. Two days later, when I went back, it was gone, but I like to think that someone took it home and it is inspiring them. I left both English and French translations of the same message, to reach as many people as possible!"

Sadie P. • 21 • Angers, France

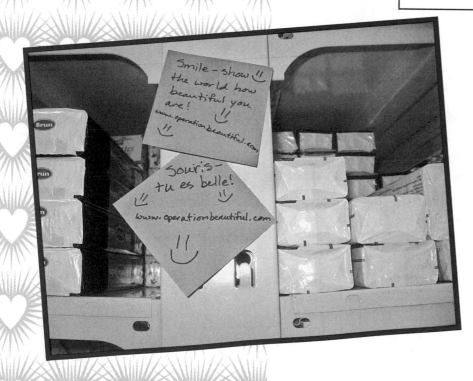

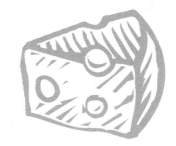

DIETING:
A SIREN'S SONG

We're a nation in love with the concept of dieting, but dieting doesn't love us back. Diets rarely deliver on their promises, and they come with a load of baggage. Falling in love with a diet can distort your views of your body, nutritional needs, and hunger cues for years to come.

Here's the real lowdown on the lure of dieting:

- Operation Beautiful uses the word "diet" to refer to low-calorie meal plans that are designed as quick fixes. Diets typically recommend cutting out an entire food group or replacing legitimate meals with foodlike substances, such as diet bars or shakes. Most diets rarely mention the importance of physical activity as a complement to their meal plan. Diets call for sudden changes in eating patterns and typically focus more on numbers (such as calories or grams of protein) than the nutritional value of the food. Although different diets claim to have found the magic "cure" for our weight woes, they all typically work by simply restricting calories, whether it's from carbohydrates, proteins, or fats. As a result, diets create drastic results, which is why many people find them appealing at first.

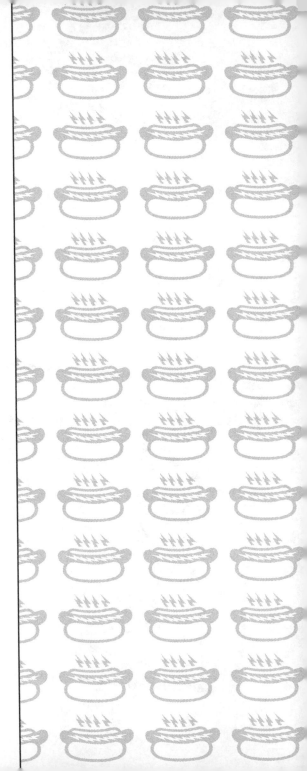

- Some eating programs (such as Weight Watchers) or online support groups (such as SparkPeople) promote a well-balanced approach to eating and an active lifestyle. These eating programs focus on sound techniques to lose weight, such as portion control, and can be useful in achieving and maintaining a healthy weight. Sensible eating programs stress moderation, as well as a slow and steady weight loss; on the other hand, diets champion restriction and quick fixes.

- Research shows that diets may be successful in the short-term; however, they rarely produce long-lasting results and are impossible to maintain for long. "Whenever I have clients tell me they're on some sort of restrictive diet, I ask if they can visualize themselves eating this way in a year, five years from now, or when they're sixty-five years old. They usually say no, and then admit to not enjoying their diet anyway!" says Janel Ovrut, R.D., who works with clients to lose weight in a healthy, maintainable manner.

- Dieting can have long-term impacts on our ability to eat according to our internal cues and without guilt. "Diets teach people not to trust their body," says Dr. Susan Albers, author of the book *Eating Mindfully: How to End Mindless Eating and Enjoy a Balanced Relationship with Food*. "Diets are about following rules rather than your hunger. For a segment of the population, diets are even dangerous. If you have a predisposition to an eating disorder, going on a diet can be a factor in triggering it."

- Dieters may believe that they are being healthy by losing weight, even if they only keep it off only for a short time. However, research has shown that yo-yo dieting (consistently losing and gaining weight) is extremely harmful, both physically and emotionally. Although there is contradictory research, some studies have shown that yo-yo dieting can lead to high blood pressure and high cholesterol. "Furthermore, losing and then regaining weight can cause one to be discouraged or feel like a failure," says Janel Ovrut, R.D. "It is more beneficial to make healthy lifestyle changes that last and have a positive effect on weight loss. Set gradual, maintainable goals for a healthy approach to weight loss, and look beyond shortcut diets."

- Diets rarely promote moderation, as strict ad-herence to a meal plan creates the most obvious and immediate results. However, extreme eating behaviors, such as avoiding entire food groups or eating a very low-calorie diet, can have serious emotional, as well as physical, consequences. "Fad diets can warp your relationship to food. For example, let's say you are on a low-carbohydrate diet. This changes your perception of foods like bread and pasta forever," says Dr. Albers. Do you really want to go through life avoiding spaghetti?

- Dieting teaches us that food is the enemy. Diets instruct us to restrict food, offering tips such as, "Drink water to feel fuller" or "Never finish all the food on your plate no matter how much is served." Also, most diets rarely focus on the nutritional value of food; instead, food simply becomes about the number of calories or grams of protein that it contains. This focus on quantity over quality can be mentally damaging and result in malnutrition of key nutrients.

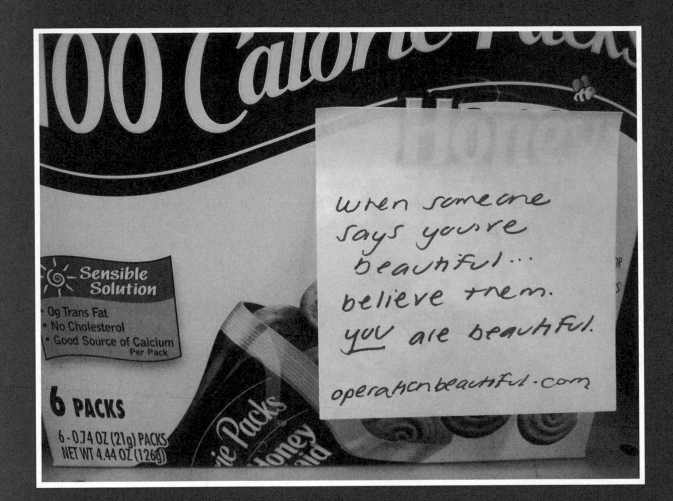

Kristen S. • 23 • Minnesota

Counting: Fuzzy Math

So many people feel out of control when it comes to their weight and their eating. One way to get that control back—or so we think—is to count. Count calories, count grams of sugar, count servings, count number of vegetables, count grams of protein. After all, weight loss is a simple math equation: If calories burned are higher than calories consumed, your body will drop excess fat. We line up the numbers after each meal, add, and then subtract from our goal number.

Something about counting appeals to a lot of women. Counting is neat; it is orderly; and it is scientific. Counting is clear and simple when so many things about dieting and weight loss are not.

For Kath Younger, counting calories helped her lose the thirty pounds she had slowly gained during college, a result of overeating and a reduction in her activity levels following foot surgery. "Throughout my weight loss and the first year of maintenance, I kept an online food diary to keep an eye on what I ate. I heartily believe (and tons of research supports) that food diaries are extremely helpful to increase awareness and accountability of food intake," says Kath, who is twenty-seven years old and studying to be a dietitian. "I think counting calories is a good idea for those seeking to lose weight because it's way too easy to eat too much in our culture. There are many ways to keep an eye on portions—Weight

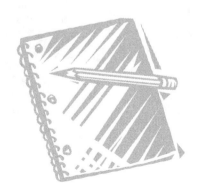

Watchers, counting food groups, counting calories, and more. In my opinion, calories are the easiest to monitor, as long as you are mindful about the balance of nutrients in your diet as well. Counting really helped me realize how easy it was to sneak in empty calories here and there and how quickly they add up."

Kath admits to being a detail-oriented person and says that the nature of calorie counting appealed to her; she was successful in counting in that she never became obsessed with the numbers. However, for many other women, calorie counting—or counting in any form—becomes a burden, not a healthy tool. Instead of using calorie counting to create balanced, portion-controlled meals like Kath did, some people find that counting becomes an obstacle to healthy eating. What happens if you're about to sit down for dinner, and there are only fifty calories "left" in your allotment for the day? What if you go for an extra-long walk around the neighborhood and need an additional snack to fuel you? What if you just don't feel hungry on a certain day—do you eat regardless of your satiety cues to meet your calorie quota?

An extreme focus on counting also diminishes the real value of food—its nutritional content. "In the beginning of my weight-loss journey, I was more focused on counting calories and not so much where the calories were coming from. I'd have a cookie or a sugary granola bar as long as it fit in," observes Kath. Food is about so much more than the number of calories it contains, and our over-reliance on counting takes our attention away from eating whole, natural foods full of the antioxidants and vitamins our bodies crave.

The craziest thing about counting is that we treat it as absolute, but it's really so abstract. We read a nutritional

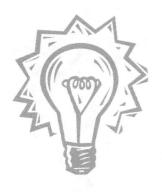

label and accept it as the truth, but maybe our half-cup scoop of oatmeal is slightly larger than it is supposed to be. We pencil in "252 calories" in our workout log because that is what the elliptical told us, but maybe we have a higher percentage of muscle mass and actually burned more. A doctor tells us we need to eat two thousand calories to maintain our current weight, so that's the goal we strive for—but how does the doctor know this is true? Each of these numbers are just approximations, and while they are helpful tools, calorie counts are not the be-all and end-all of dieting, weight-loss success, or maintenance. Calorie counting is just fuzzy math.

Furthermore, calorie counting on a day-to-day basis disregards the fact that our bodies do not magically reset themselves every twenty-four hours. Whether we lose, gain, or maintain our weight is not determined on how many calories we eat in a given meal; our weight is the result of many days of meals and workouts. Some days, we may eat more food because we meet up with a friend for a dinner out. The next day, we might not need as much fuel because we took the day off from exercising. A consequence of calorie counting is that we learn not to trust our bodies and hunger and satiety cues; we may become too reliant on what the numbers tell us to do and not do.

"The more I read about health and nutrition, the more I realized that the numbers just don't matter. As clichéd as it sounds, it is about how you feel on the inside that matters most. As long as I was putting in the effort to eat the right foods and keep on exercising, I didn't care what number the scale came back with," says Kath. "It took about a year of maintaining my weight loss to feel confident in my ability to make good judgments in portions and balance."

"During my college years, I struggled with my body image and how many calories I consumed in a day. Looking back, I can't believe I put my beautiful body through hell for four to five years. These notes from Operation Beautiful inspire me to appreciate my body more and more every day and not to worry about how many calories I consumed in a day. Be beautiful in who you are and be grateful for the curves you've got because you only get one body. If you screw it up, you can't go back and fix it."

Kristen G. • 27 • Fairfield, Connecticut

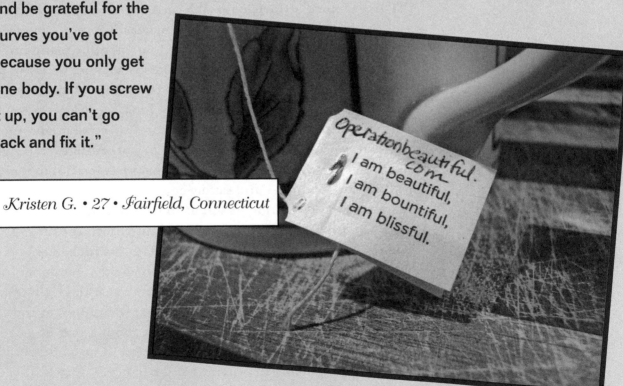

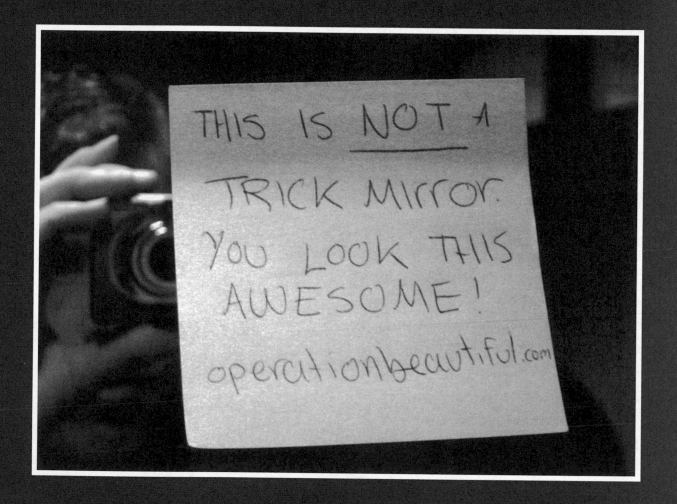

B. A. Coyne • 22 • Vancouver,
British Columbia, Canada

"When I was sixteen years old, I began making myself throw up. One day, I had eaten with one of my best friends and afterward, I ran to the bathroom. When I was finished, I opened the door to find my best friend standing on the other side in tears. She was so mad at me. She said that if I didn't confess to my dad, she would tell him herself. I knew she would do it (she was a good friend!), and deep down, I knew what I was doing was bad for me. Later, I told my dad while I was at the doctor's office. I thought he would be so mad, and I was so scared to tell him. But when I told him what I had been doing to myself, he started to cry and just hugged me. He told me he loved me, I was beautiful, and he would get me help. At this point I was glad that I had come clean, but I didn't really want help. I wasn't 'done' yet. I still felt fat; I was still unhappy with myself.

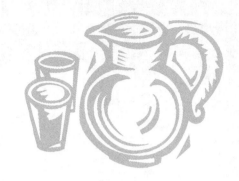

Kristen • 29 • Ottawa, Ontario, Canada

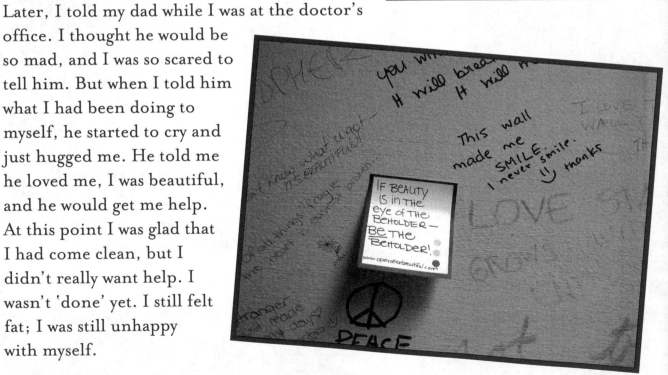

178

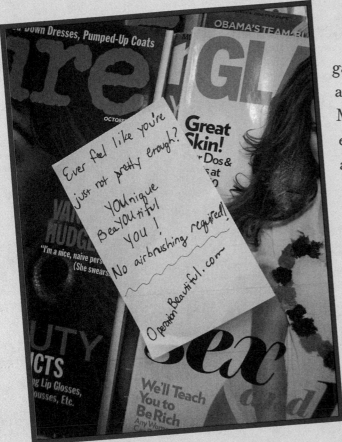

On the note in the image:
"Ever feel like you're just not pretty enough?

YOUnique
BeaYOUtiful
YOU!

No airbrushing required!

OperationBeautiful.com"

Jana P. • 46 • Garland, Texas

After college, I got married and had gained a lot of weight. I wanted to make a change. I joined Weight Watchers in May 2007. It was the best move I have ever made. I lost seventy-five pounds and have kept it off. Now I know how to eat healthy and make positive food choices, and I use food for fuel and not an emotional crutch.

I think that girls need to learn the difference between their diet and dieting. I am a firm believer that your diet is what you eat every day—not what you do to lose weight. I hate fad diets, 1,200-calorie diets, and salad-only diets. We are human, and we have cravings, lifestyle changes, and desires to try new things. One of my favorite things to do is to turn yummy but unhealthy recipes into something [healthier] that I feel good about putting into my body."

Tatum Hernandez • 24 •
Marion, Ohio

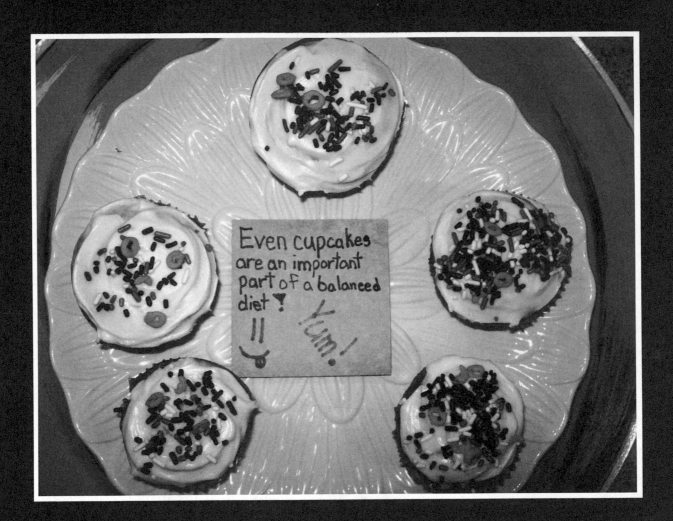

Emily Filostrat • 15 • Virginia

"Yesterday, I was in The Gap. I went in the fitting room, locked the door, and held up a pair of jeans in front of me. Looking in the mirror, I thought to myself, 'These are not going to fit.' I already started to feel the negative talk start building up. Immediately, I imagined that that same mirror I was staring at had an Operation Beautiful note on it and what it said! Needless to say, it nipped those negative thoughts I was having and I felt better right away!"

Krista Wehrer • 30 • Santa Rosa, California

"I am so over scales. Last year, I weighed myself at least once a week and that drove me nuts. Then, I didn't weigh myself at all from June to mid-October. When I finally did, I was completely fine with the number because I realized it didn't mean a damn thing. I like the way I look, I fit into my clothes, I'm healthier than ever, and I'm happier than ever. I wish all women would give the scales a break for several months at a time, especially if they're addicted to the numbers. Because that's all they are—symbols to represent a quantity. A number should never measure self-worth, value, or happiness."

Kailey Harless • 22 • Athens, Ohio

"I started participating in Operation Beautiful because I have had low self-esteem in the past. The first note I posted was in the gym at Arizona State University's West Campus. Every day I see girls of all shapes and sizes in the gym, and they are all so beautiful! I posted this note in the morning when I put my gym bag away and was hoping all day that when I came back later, it would still be up. Much to my surprise, it was! I was sitting down putting on my shoes when I saw a girl walking out of the bathroom with it. She walked up to her friend and said, 'Look! Look what someone put on the mirror!' I had the biggest smile on my face——it was the best day I had had in a long time. Every woman should know just how beautiful she is, inside and out!"

Courtney Murch • 22 • Mesa, Arizona

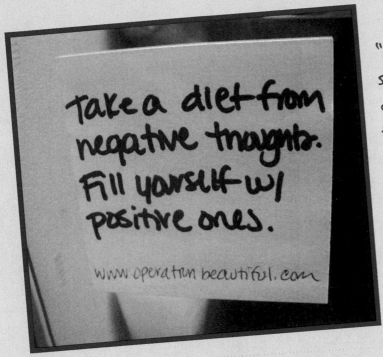

take a diet from negative thoughts. Fill yourself w/ positive ones.

www.operationbeautiful.com

Michelle Gay • 26 • Australia

"I used to weigh myself obsessively, and I became so focused on every little fluctuation that it completely controlled my life. I would count every calorie, every day. I weigh myself about once a month now. Otherwise, I go by the way I feel and look in the mirror. Before, I often found that I felt I looked better before I weighed myself and then totally beat myself up for every imperfection after getting off the scale. I realized that that behavior was so toxic for me that I didn't need to obsess over it . . . and mainly because of Operation Beautiful."

Kristy Cox • 24 • Charleston, South Carolina

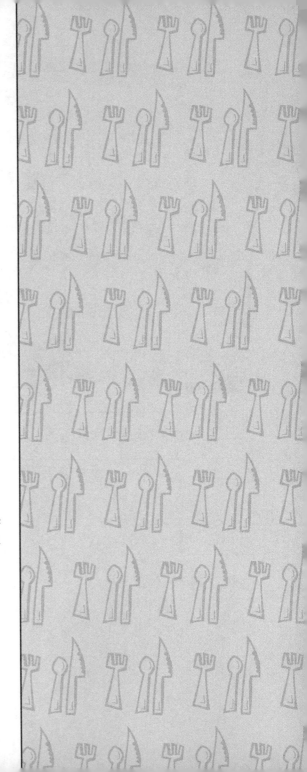

THE DIETLESS DIET

You may be wondering, "If diets don't work, and constantly counting is too tiresome, how am I going to reach or stay at a healthy weight?" Believe it or not, you don't have to spend the rest of your life in a cycle of yo-yo diets. You can free yourself of the obsession with food. Forget about restricting yourself, and stop feeling guilty for the occasional indulgence. Get off the diet merry-go-round; it's time to live a life of balance. It sounds crazy, but it works!

- The Dietless Diet is the opposite of a fad diet: It's not restrictive or drastic. The Dietless Diet focuses on eating real, natural foods—not packaged, processed foodlike substances—in reasonable portions. It works because you listen to your hunger cues—on the Dietless Diet, you eat when you are hungry, and you stop when you are full. Best of all, this way of eating allows you to enjoy the occasional indulgent meal or dessert. When you eat balanced, nutritious meals 90 percent of the time, you don't need to obsess over a delicious slice of chocolate cake.

- The next time you're at the grocery store, flip over that package of cookies, macaroni and cheese, cereal, or deli meat and read the ingredient list.

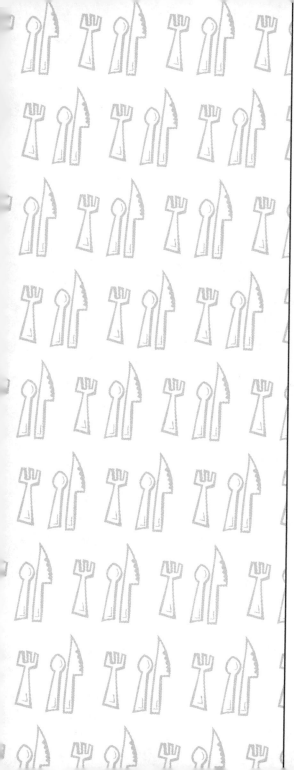

On diets, we tend to just focus on the numbers—how many calories or how much protein. But on the Dietless Diet, we're more concerned with the quality of the foods we put in our mouth. How many ingredients are in those crackers? Can you pronounce most of them? Were the ingredients created in a laboratory or grown in the ground? Filling your grocery cart with real food—like lean meat, fish, beans, brown rice, oatmeal, sweet potatoes, green peppers, apples, skim milk, and eggs—is a smart move because these products are typically lower in calories than processed foods and better for your body, too. "The simple answer to our weight woes is to eat more whole foods and less processed foods, and eat in moderation," says Dr. Carolyn Becker.

- Eat more plants! "Americans get most of their excessive dietary fat and calories through animal products," notes Dr. Denise Martz. Fill up your plate with veggies and fruits, which are typically low-calorie, high-fiber foods that promote satiety without breaking the caloric bank. Vegetables don't have to be a boring side dish; try coating broccoli in a little extra virgin oil olive, Parmesan cheese, and pepper and roasting it in the oven until browned. Alternatively, sneak some grilled zucchini or steamed spinach into your regular pasta dishes—you won't even notice the veggies are there! If you're feeling brave, try tossing a handful of fresh spinach into your regular fruit smoothies. The green color might throw you off, but the taste is virtually undetectable.

- Make it easy to eat well. Keep your fridge and pantry stocked with healthy options so you're less likely to eat out. Prepare and freeze lunches and dinners (like casseroles) on Sunday night to fuel you through the week. "I recommend to my clients that they chop up their produce upon bringing it home from the grocery store and put it in clear Tupperware containers on the top shelf," says Janel Ovrut, R.D. "You can also leave cut-up fruit and veggies out on the kitchen table for the family to snack on throughout the day. Having healthy, appealing foods at the ready makes eating nutritious foods much more accessible and enjoyable."

- On the Dietless Diet, it's important to take pleasure in eating by sitting down at the table and focusing on your meal. "Take mindful bites," says Dr. Susan Albers. "Really enjoy your food. When you eat mindlessly, you can eat an entire plate of food and not taste one bite." Pay attention to the smell, taste, texture, and temperature of your food. Try to chew it more thoroughly instead of just slamming food down your throat. When we do not eat mindfully, we are more likely to overeat and less likely to feel satisfied by our food, no matter how healthy or delicious it is.

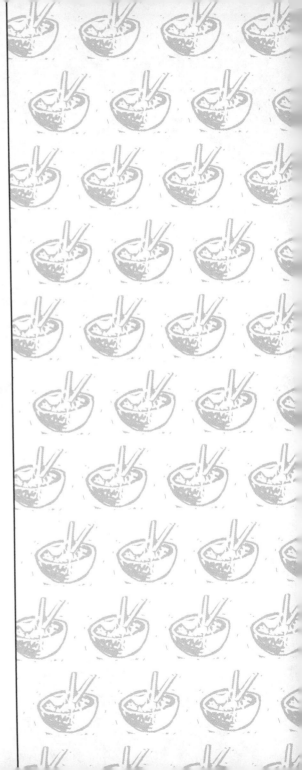

- Listen to your body's natural cues to determine if you're really hungry or if you're just tempted to eat out of boredom, sadness, joy, or simply because it's "time to eat." It can be difficult to hear your body's cues after years of yo-yo dieting; however, regaining the ability to tell whether you are truly hungry or full is the key to losing or maintaining weight without restricting foods. Activities such as yoga or meditation can help you feel more in touch with your body's cues.

- Also, pay close attention to how food makes you feel. After switching to the whole, natural Dietless Diet, you may notice that you feel less tired, suffer from fewer headaches, and have a longer attention span than you did when eating processed, gimmicky diet foods. "We've become so detached from what we're putting into our bodies," says Janel Ovrut, R.D. "We often fail to realize that every last bit of food we put into our bodies has a direct effect on our health." Reinforce how great eating well makes you feel, and you'll be more likely to reach for an apple for your afternoon snack than a bag of chips.

- On the Dietless Diet, there is no reason to freak out after one calorie-rich meal, as you have been practicing moderation and balance for 90 percent of your meals. It's important to take a macro view of your eating habits and strive to find balance in the big picture. If you're tempted to overeat and feel out of control in your decision to indulge, try to stop the unhealthy behavior before it starts by going for a walk, brushing your teeth, drinking a cup of tea, or finding another way to distract yourself from the urge to binge. Also, analyze why you're tempted to overeat, which is often triggered by an unprocessed emotion, such as sadness or boredom.

· If you're unsure about portion sizes or other aspects of healthy eating, consider making an appointment with a registered dietitian. A dietitian will work with you to form a clear, concise plan for your new lifestyle.

· Cut through the media hype about what to eat, and educate yourself so you're more equipped to make healthy choices. Books such as *In Defense of Food* by Michael Pollan and *Food Matters: A Guide to Conscious Eating* by Mark Bittman are excellent resources that provide a balanced, commonsense approach to eating in the real world. *Intuitive Eating: A Revolutionary Program That Works* by Evelyn Tribole and Elyse Resch provides a wealth of information on mindful eating.

When Food Is the Enemy

Sophia hates it when people ask her, "So, when did this all start? Why did you become anorexic?" The questions bother her because they imply that she chose to develop an eating disorder, like it's a hobby or an extracurricular activity. "It's as if they believe there was one, single moment of decision when I made up my mind to become anorexic," says Sophia, a twenty-two-year-old from Los Angeles. "But that's not how anorexia is. I definitely did not choose anorexia, nor did I foresee the nearly unbreakable control it would hold over me."

In the United States, ten million females suffer from anorexia or bulimia—more than the number of women afflicted with breast cancer. More than four million Americans suffer from binge-eating disorder. Millions more suffer in silence, undiagnosed and struggling every day. It's not just an issue for women, either; one out of every ten people suffering from an eating disorder is male.

Sophia's battle with her eating disorder began more than five years ago, and she believes it was triggered by her lack of self-esteem, envy of other women, and drive for perfectionism. When combined, Sophia says these qualities were a recipe for disaster. "I slowly, gradually got sucked into the vortex of disordered eating. I counted calories. I avoided social events that had to do with food. I started reading up on diet books, looking at pictures of models for 'thinspiration.' And day by day, I fed my eating disorder with continuous negative thoughts and developed disordered habits until it turned into a full-fledged obsession," she remembers. "Over my senior year of high school, I lost so much weight that my guidance counselor called my parents in for a talk. She suggested that I might have an eating disorder. I vehemently denied it. She made me get on a scale, and I was disgustingly thin—just seventy-four pounds with heavy winter clothing on. There was nothing more I could say."

Sophia's parents hospitalized her, but after five days, she sought her own release against doctor's orders. While her parents tried to help, she says she simply wasn't "ready" to give up her eating disorder, turning to bulimia as a new way to control her weight and emotions. The years passed, but Sophia felt as if she wasn't really living. "I was obsessed with every meal, every morsel that touched my lips, and after a meal, I was already thinking about the next meal," she says. "I was terribly unhappy, lonely, and depressed."

Recovery came slowly and in a surprising way. A man with a mental disorder at Sophia's church asked if someone would help him read the Bible, and Sophia volunteered. "He didn't have an eating disorder, but he did have a lot of characteristics that all mentally disordered people share: obsessive behaviors, irrational thoughts and habits, inability to socialize, and totally neglected and misunderstood by society," she remembers. "I don't know why, but when I heard that he needed help, I suddenly felt a strong pang of pity and empathy, so I volunteered to teach him." It must have been a strange sight, Sophia admits. "A too-thin girl, teaching a thirty-three-year-old man to read the Bible . . . but we shared a special connection because we were both hopeless, dejected, mentally deceived people. That was when I started to clearly see how freaking *evil* this mental disorder is. As I heard him talk about his fears and anxieties, it was so, so crazy, but the worst part was that those feelings were so like my own crazy thoughts and behaviors." At that point, Sophia says she truly started to detest her eating disorder and tried to move forward.

A few months later, Sophia joined her parents on a mission

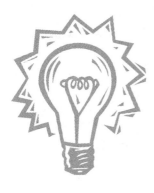

trip in Southeast Asia. While in a foreign country with strange foods, Sophia's eating disorder had nowhere to hide. "I was totally forced out of my comfort zone. If you've ever been out of the country, you'll understand—there is no country in the world with as many diet products as America. Those foods were just not readily available in Singapore," Sophia says. The experience also forced her to get out of her house, socialize with friends, and attend church with greater frequency. "At first, I was freaking out. But the more I started challenging myself, the easier and easier it got as time went by."

Every eating disorder story is different. Each woman—or man—can recall a different trigger to their unhealthy behaviors. Some struggle to eat; some struggle to stop eating. Some seek out professional help; some turn to friends. Some eating disorders fade gently with time and treatment, and others rage on for many years. The people that achieve recovery find it in many different ways. Some find recovery at a treatment center; some find their own way out of the darkness with the support of family; others find it in an Operation Beautiful note.

But everyone with an eating disorder has one thing in common—the need to hope. Hold on to the hope that things can change. You must put in the work; you must have the desire to get past it. But know that you can do it. "Hope is your lifeline. During recovery, you are bound to meet some failures. But never give up, and never hate yourself for it," says Sophia. "Recovery is not an exponential upward increase but an overall and gradual upward climb. Relish each victory you make, and use it as more encouragement to push you further toward recovery. Recovery is possible, and the result is well worth it."

"For almost two years, I've been battling with food and weight demons. I feel divided and split in two. I can see that ditching half of my lunch in the bin in the morning to prevent myself from eating it later is irrational, and that I can safely eat the food without gaining weight, but I do it anyway. I know that a spoonful of butter in my mashed potatoes isn't going to kill me, but it doesn't stop me from throwing it away from me like a bottle full of arsenic. It's a clear fact that my weight is too low for my height and age, but it doesn't stop me from panicking every time the scales hitch up a pound, and doesn't stop me from cutting down on what I eat for the rest of the day. Eating disorders aren't always about being thin or looking good. It started that way for me, but nowadays, it really isn't."

"*There is NO such thing as PERFECTION! Embrace your IMPERFECTIONS & LOVE YOURSELF!*"

Kirsten • 22 • Wichita, Kansas

Francesca • 15 • England

192

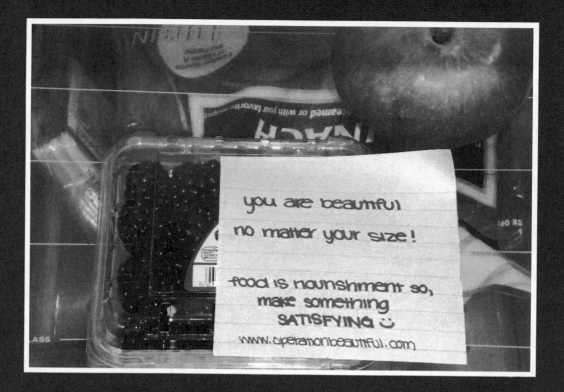

you are beautiful
no matter your size!

food is nourishment so,
make something
SATISFYING :)
www.operationbeautiful.com

"After three years of recovery from an eating disorder, I am finally at a place where food doesn't scare me. I eat my

Jacquie • 23 • Washington, Đ.C.

meals and snacks in order to fuel my busy schedule of classes, an internship, and fun with friends. I don't starve myself in order to be the 'perfect person' and do not feel the urge to binge and purge in order to express my feelings. I keep a note in my refrigerator to remind myself that food is not my enemy and no matter what the number on the scale says or the number inside my clothes is, it's okay. It's beautiful. My health is beautiful."

"I dealt with anorexia nervosa off and on for four years—from when I was sixteen until I was twenty. Looking back, I wish that I hadn't given over such a big part of my life to my disorder.

A huge step in my recovery came when I became a resident assistant winter quarter of my junior year. I knew that as an RA, I needed to be seen as strong, and by not eating, I was not strong and was destroying my body and my life. I wanted to set a good example, and wanted to be there for my residents when they needed me. But, the day that I decided that I was no longer the girl with the eating disorder was a day not long after I started dating my boyfriend. We had been together three weeks or so at the time, and were headed into the dining hall for dinner. At that time, I realized that I didn't want him to see me as weird—I wanted to be normal. I wanted to be normal for my family, my boy-friend, and especially myself. On that day, I knew that I was going to cast away my eating disorder and start living my

Crystal Newberry • 28 •
Toronto, Ontario, Canada

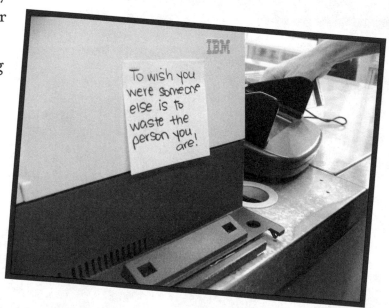

To wish you were someone else is to waste the person you are!

194

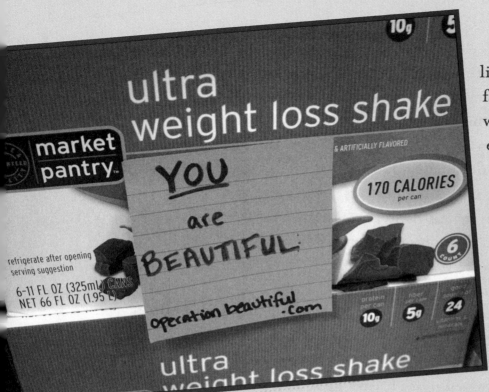

Jess Furrow • 24 •
Grand Rapids, Michigan

life to its fullest. That fateful day in June, I walked away from my eating disorder.

For people who are still struggling with disordered eating patterns, I think the biggest thing that you can do for yourself is ask for help. Asking for help can be the first step to recovery, and it shows that you are stronger than the eating disorder, regardless of what the disorder tells you. Recovery goes beyond learning normal eating habits, and having someone to talk to was instrumental for my recovery. There are so many people in your life who are ready to listen and to help you with whatever you may need to find recovery. An eating disorder is not normal, but you can break away from its hold and be the person that you were meant to be."

Deva S. • 23 • Cincinnati, Ohio

"I struggled with binge eating and bulimia in the past, but I've successfully kept off seventy pounds for the last two years—the healthy way. I think the primary reason I've been successful is that I've been able to take the long view when it comes to my health. I want to have a family in the future and be a positive healthy role model for my kids. I can see myself running a marathon with my husband and kids cheering from the sidelines, and it really motivates me. My parents were both overweight when I was growing up, and their bad habits and negative self-image (especially my mom's) made a strong impression on me and how I see myself. I don't want to do the same thing to my kids. I've also been working very hard at eliminating guilt and regret from my life, especially when it comes to food and exercise. It isn't productive to beat myself up for eating something 'bad.' Plus, the guilt tends to lead to more bingeing, followed by even more guilt, and eventually by purging, if the binge was really big. I'm trying to avoid binges before they start now, by really processing why I feel the need to binge. More often than not I want to binge because I'm stressed or upset, and I can make myself feel better by working out, writing, talking to a friend, taking the dog for a walk, or a million other things that aren't food."

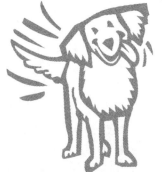

Kara • 26 • New York, New York

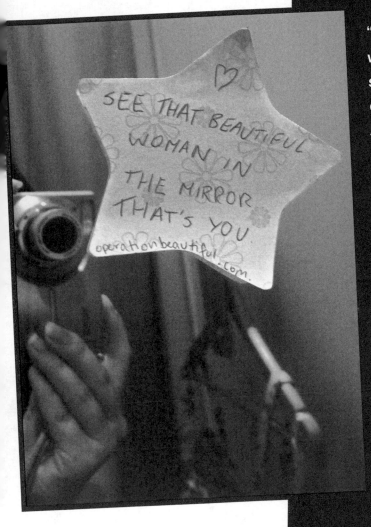

"I may not be perfect, but I see myself for what I am—beautiful and unique. When I stumbled upon Operation Beautiful, I was ecstatic and immediately wanted to help. Armed with a stack of Post-its, a camera, and a few inspiring words, my little sister and I set off for a day in the city. Surprisingly, it turned out to be the most fun we've ever had in the city. Tayla would stand watch as I'd hastily scribble out notes and paste them to mirrors, books, walls, and store windows. Trying to keep our anonymity whilst posting gave us a thrill, and the warm feeling we got from knowing we could have made someone happy lingered for days. It alarms me just how many amazing, smart, and gorgeous women Fat Talk themselves into thinking they're ugly. I'm so glad that I can help women regain their good body image, and that I can make sure that my little sister keeps hers."

Ashleigh Ubank • 20 • Brisbane, Queensland, Australia

UNIQUE

You are valuable
I am a ... I personality? With an unu...
I AM a! ♥ my curves + highlight I HAVE a
This is me... woman
I feel intense... you are so
people are much more than
you are so much more than your looks!
you look! your looks!
you are healthy
I'm in synk with who i am

Your face lights up when you SMILE

I am compassion kindness loving Confident Strong
I have a good smile brighten up a room & make you smile

Go Rockies!

Special

You have inherent value; worth
You have such an amazing personality!
You rock in that outfit
I AM Beautiful

Joyful
worth it
I am! just the way i am! I love myself Powerful

Your hair shines so prettily!

You have style

Your eyes Sparkle
You have stunning
You are comfortable...
You have comfortable in your clothes
You're smile warms my heart
You stand w/ Confidence

"I am in a program for eating disorders. During our body image class, we made a runway. First, we wrote down the negative comments we say to ourselves about our bodies—body bashing. The therapists walked down the runway, and we had to call out everything we had written down. It felt so mean to say these things that we say to ourselves every day to someone else. We then flipped the runway over and wrote down positive body affirmations, like how much we love what our body does for us. We then each took a turn walking down the runway while everyone else said the positive affirmations that were written down out loud. It was a great experience. Think about what a better world we would live in if we swapped out saying all the negatives for the positives. You wouldn't say those horrible negative body image comments to someone else; why say them to yourself? Love your body, love yourself."

Rachel C. • 19 • Denver, Colorado

Loosening the Grip

It is possible to free yourself from an eating disorder, but in order to be successful, you must approach recovery with knowledge and purpose. It's important to understand why you've gotten to this point, how you can begin to heal your relationship with your body and food, and why you want to recover in the first place.

It's easy to feel like no one understands what you are going through. Your friends may shy away; your significant other might say the wrong things; your parents may fight with you at the dinner table. Take comfort in the fact that you're not alone, and there is hope. Millions of other women have been where you are now, and they've come out on the other side, stronger than ever.

To help you on your journey, here is the best real-life advice from women in recovery:

- Admitting that you need help is very important. Professional treatment will help you cope with the mental, emotional, and physical ramifications of an eating disorder. In-patient treatment facilities are the most effective forms of therapy, but they are often not covered by insurance. If you're a student, you may have access to free therapy sessions at your high school or college. Many churches and temples offer free therapy to members. Also, search the Internet for self-help groups in your area, but verify they are led by a professional before attending. Your local or state government may also provide discounted therapy; ask your therapist for details.

• Stop living in secret, and tell someone about your eating disorder. Convey how serious the situation is and that you need help. "Try to get over the shame and the embarrassment, and talk to someone you trust about it. Once it's out in the open, it suddenly becomes so much easier to think about overcoming it," says Anna W., a twenty-six-year-old who struggled with bulimia for eight years, beginning when she was a sophomore in high school.

• Also, recognize that your family and friends may have their own personal limitations that may prevent them from helping you in a healthy, productive way. "My family tried to be helpful, but they did the exact opposite," says Morgan, a twenty-five-year-old in Illinois who struggled with anorexia, purging, and over-exercising. "They were always commenting on how I looked instead of how I felt." When dealing with someone who is insensitive, consider where they are coming from: Do they have their own issues with food, weight, or self-esteem? Do they have trouble connecting emotionally with others? Do they feel your situation may be their fault?

- Discover what the eating disorder is really about and deal with those issues. Many women who have eating disorders can trace the cause back to self-esteem issues, personality factors, childhood or adult trauma, job/career pressures, or other life-altering situations. Dealing with the issue behind your eating disorder (possibly with the assistance of a therapist) is pivotal to the recovery process.

- Process your emotions instead of burying them inside your eating disorder. Try to find positive outlets, such as writing in your diary or a blog, practicing yoga, or calling a close friend, whenever you feel the need to use your eating disorder as a crutch.

- Refocus your energies into a new hobby—find a new skill to learn or rediscover an old passion. "My anorexia had a way of making me believe that I was not worth putting time or energy into. As I started to recover, I rediscovered who I was. I found that I enjoy chalk pastels, collages, music therapy, writing, bead work, painting my nails, and bubble baths," says Jessica Daly, a twenty-four-year-old from Allentown, Pennsylvania. "Every time that I choose to do something for myself, I refuse the disorder and choose life instead of death. Finding the authentic real me has been the biggest joy in my life today." For Kara K., a twenty-six-year-old who was diagnosed with anorexia as a teenager, taking martial arts classes helped advance her recovery. "Tae Kwon Do and kung fu helped me realize the need for good fuel and gave me an outlet for stress," she says.

• Face reality: Consider what you want out of your life and how much your eating disorder has cost you. Has your eating disorder made you any happier? Has it furthered your career or education goals? Or has your eating disorder wasted your time and energy, ruined opportunities, and destroyed relationships?

• Realize that you may never be 100 percent free from your struggle with your eating disorder. The knowledge that you must stay aware of any creeping distorted thoughts or behaviors is very powerful. "There are days when I look in the mirror and cannot stand what I see," admits Jessica S., a twenty-one-year-old from Spartanburg, South Carolina, who battled undiagnosed anorexia in high school. "I think all of these thoughts, and then I snap myself out of it by thinking about all of the things my body can do—it's amazing. In general, as women, we have our days when we hate how we look, which is normal. It's not normal having those thoughts take over our lives, which is something that only those who have experienced can fully understand."

- Remember that recovery is a choice you must actively make. "There are no easy answers or quick fixes, but I think of recovery as a choice—I cruise through some days without a moment's hesitation, and I have days when I constantly have to make that conscious choice," says Ellie, a twenty-seven-year-old from the United Kingdom who was hospitalized for anorexia. "I've learned, above all, that when you finally pluck up the courage to face the things you are most afraid of, you find out that you had the strength all along."

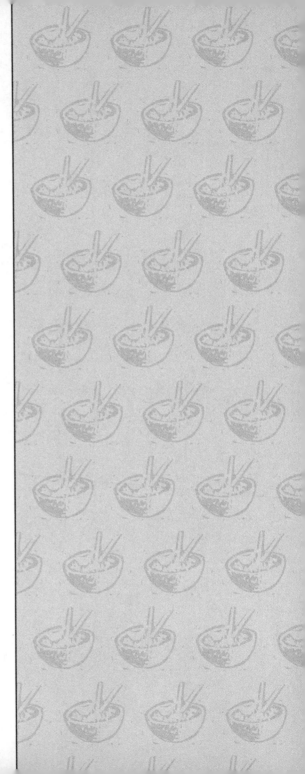

Chapter 6

Faith

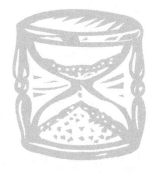

From the Trivial to the Pivotal

We worry too much about tiny things outside of our control.

By anyone's standards, Stephanie Kiehart is a beautiful woman. She has intensely green eyes and perfectly coiffed light blond hair that just barely brushes her shoulders. Stephanie wears her hair in so many different styles— blow-dried straight, neatly braided, decorated with clips or pins, wrapped in a bun, pulled into a low ponytail—that it's hard to imagine her completely bald.

The symptoms were mysterious and scary. First, she gained ten pounds. As a typical college student, she spent her weekends partying with friends, so Stephanie initially tried to halt the strange weight gain by cutting back on extra sweets and drinks. Nothing worked. "There was no apparent reason for the weight gain," remembers Stephanie. When she broke out in full body hives, she knew it was time to see a doctor—something was seriously wrong.

"Many doctors misdiagnosed me, and finally, one

discovered a ten-pound tumor on my ovary," she says. "When I was cut open on the operating table, the doctors realized it was cancerous, and it was everywhere." When Stephanie woke up from the anesthesia, she was told the cancer was in her appendix, bladder, right ovary, and all the lymph nodes in her lower abdomen. She was only twenty-one years old, and she was facing stage 3C ovarian cancer.

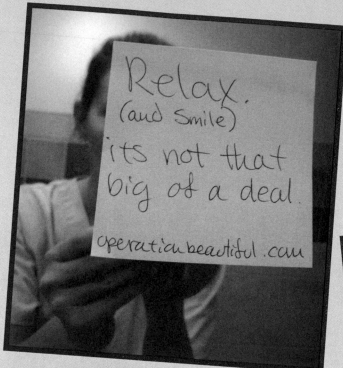

Relax.
(and smile)
its not that
big of a deal.

operationbeautiful.com

Her doctors recommended that Stephanie begin chemotherapy immediately, and Stephanie took a leave of absence from college to receive the aggressive treatment. "I was only awake for one hour a day; I lost all my hair; and I was bound to a wheelchair. I received so many shots and transfusions," she says. Her family watched in horror as the treatment made Stephanie incredibly nauseous. She began to lose weight rapidly. "Even though I was so sick, I insisted the doctors keep up the aggressive treatment. I demanded they stay on schedule."

One morning, Stephanie woke up and brushed her pretty blond hair out of her eyes with a yawn. A big clump fell out into her hands. Spurred into action, she took a trimmer to her scalp and shaved it all off in one clean buzz cut. "I couldn't sit around and watch it fall out," she admits. Her shiny, blond hair was gone, but Stephanie barely thought twice about the loss. "When you're as sick as I was, you don't really care what you look like."

Can you imagine how it feels to be deathly ill, to lose your hair, to drop out of school, to wonder if the disease will win? Imagine all the things that would seem unimportant in the face of a life-threatening disease. So many of us lose our temper over traffic jams, freak out when the grocery bill is too high, and cry in the dressing room when our bathing suit doesn't fit just so. We worry too much about tiny things outside of our control. We criticize ourselves for not being perfect at school or work. We pick fights with the people that love us the most. In short, we focus on the trivial, not the pivotal. Stephanie admits that she used to live like that, too.

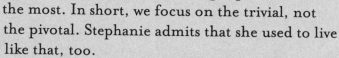

For Stephanie, cancer changed everything. "I thought about all the things I could still do—and would do again—when I was sick. Every day, I would wake up and think, 'Things will be okay. I still have both of my arms. I can still walk. I still have my family.' Even if I had been kicked out of college or lost my car, it wouldn't have mattered to me," she says. "Never for one minute did I think I was not going to make it."

Now in remission for more than five years, Stephanie realizes that cancer gave her more than it took away. "Cancer really makes you realize what you can do without. In some ways, it was an awesome experience," she admits. More than anything, her disease taught her not to sweat the small stuff. "I still close my eyes and try to get that feeling back. When things get terrible at my job or in my personal life, I realize that anything is easy after surviving chemotherapy."

Stephanie Kiehart • 26 •
Alexandria, Virginia

"Greetings from Iraq! I decided that the lovely ladies I serve with in my unit here in Iraq needed to be part of this, so I added this note to the mirror on our bathroom at work. I think everyone knew that I posted the note (there aren't many females in the unit, I am rather tall, and the note was posted at the top of the mirror!), but it stayed up until I left. The bathroom was cleaned twice a week, and the marines left it up. It is

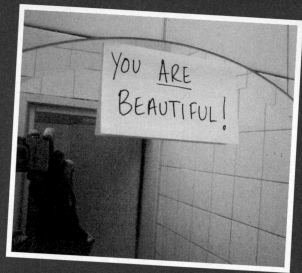

easy to forget to feel good about yourself when you are deployed with tons of men. I love this idea and plan on continuing to do this now that I'm back in the States!"

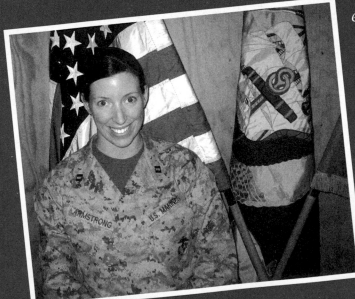

Sarah Armstrong • 31 •
Carlsbad, California

"I remember distinctly the day that my understanding of my own beauty switched from external standards (like media and comparing myself to others) to a much deeper profound appreciation stemming from the inside. I was fifteen years old, and I just got home from the gym and was crying on the washroom floor over how big I felt my butt was. Something very deep inside me said 'this isn't worth it.' It was my 'aha!' moment. I realized all the effort and energy I was putting into basically hating myself was really just spinning me in circles. It wasn't helping my life; it wasn't creating any joy; it was just making me exhausted and insecure. I really had my focus backward in

Rachael Van Rijn • 23 • Ottawa, Ontario, Canada

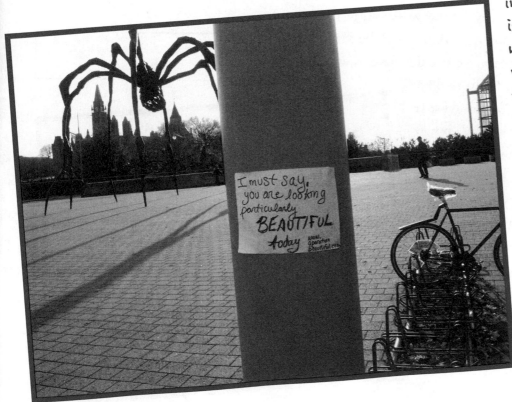

I must say, you are looking particularly BEAUTIFUL today

www. operation Beautiful.com

211

seeing what was apparently wrong instead of seeing the beauty in what I did have, like, for example, amazing red hair, beautiful curves, healthy skin, and gorgeous eyes.

I decided that really it is my own opinion that should influence how I feel about myself. In retrospect, the driving force for me wanting to lose weight was largely influenced by society, which, if left unexamined with a critical eye, has the capacity to tear down any woman's appreciation for her natural form. In line with this train of thought, I decided to stop giving so much attention to music videos, magazines, and trends. I thought to myself that I would be the most beautiful if I really let my inner self shine through and not try so hard to be what I call 'mainstream beauty.'

Those things that make us unique—like being tall and having red hair—aren't in the slightest bit bad; in fact, they should be celebrated. I decided to be an ally with myself, not an enemy."

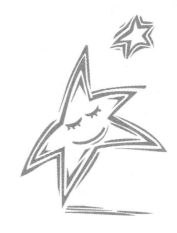

Taylor K. • 23 • Omaha, Nebraska

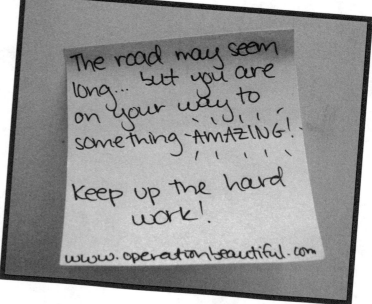

The road may seem long... but you are on your way to something AMAZING!

keep up the hard work!

www.operationbeautiful.com

212

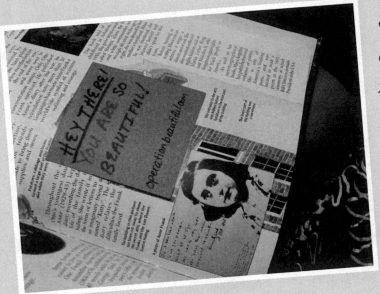

"My best friend and I decided to place this encouraging note in a book beside a picture of Anne Frank because I know she would have liked Operation Beautiful, and because I see her as a role model. She is important to me; very real and relatable, which are qualities I see Operation Beautiful giving back to girls. Every time we put a Post-it somewhere, we kiss it. Our love and support is forever a part of those notes."

Taylor H. • 15 • Illinois

"I have always been overweight and uncomfortable with how I look. I am a shy person and only talk to someone if he or she talks to me first. I am learning that this is no way to live, and I should not be afraid of what others think of me or of what I say. I am starting to realize that I have a lot to offer and that I am smart, beautiful, funny, and caring to those around me. Thank you, Operation Beautiful, for opening my eyes so that I could see the true me and start loving me for who and what I am!"

Stefanie S. • 26 • Margate, New Jersey

"When I learned about Operation Beautiful, I immediately wrote, 'Your imperfections are what make you beautiful!' on a Post-it and put it on one of the bathroom mirrors at work. It stayed up for a week. Since then, I carry my book of sticky notes with me almost everywhere.

I have found that, since I have started doing this, I am a lot more forgiving of my own imperfections. I have a big scar down the front of my leg from knee surgery. I have giant, big toes. I hate my side profile; anytime I see a picture of it I cringe. But there's nothing I can do about it. Operation Beautiful has made me a kinder person—both to others as I try to brighten someone's day with a note, as well as to myself as I begin accepting the things about me that I may not like but cannot change. I'm beautiful just the way I am, and my imperfections are what make me beautiful."

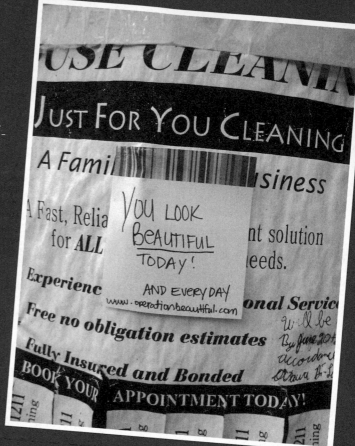

Kristen • 29 • Ottawa, Ontario, Canada

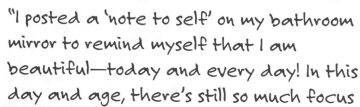

"I posted a 'note to self' on my bathroom mirror to remind myself that I am beautiful—today and every day! In this day and age, there's still so much focus on being skinny enough to fit into 'skinny jeans' and fitting the fashion industry's notion of what is beautiful. I am not a size two, nor will I ever be. I am a size ten—the perfect ten, you may say! It's taken me a while to get to the point that I can say it and believe it—and I believe it's been with the help of Operation Beautiful! I just want to be happy and healthy."

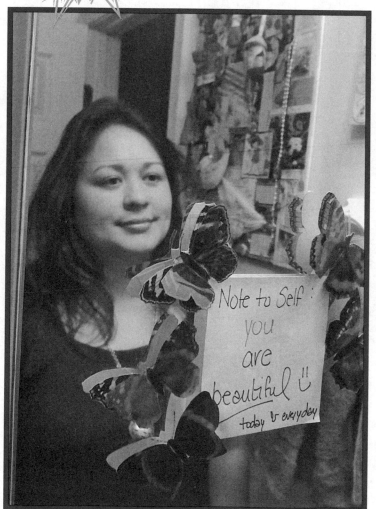

Note to Self: you are beautiful :) today & everyday

Wilma Parks • 34 • Outer Banks, North Carolina

215

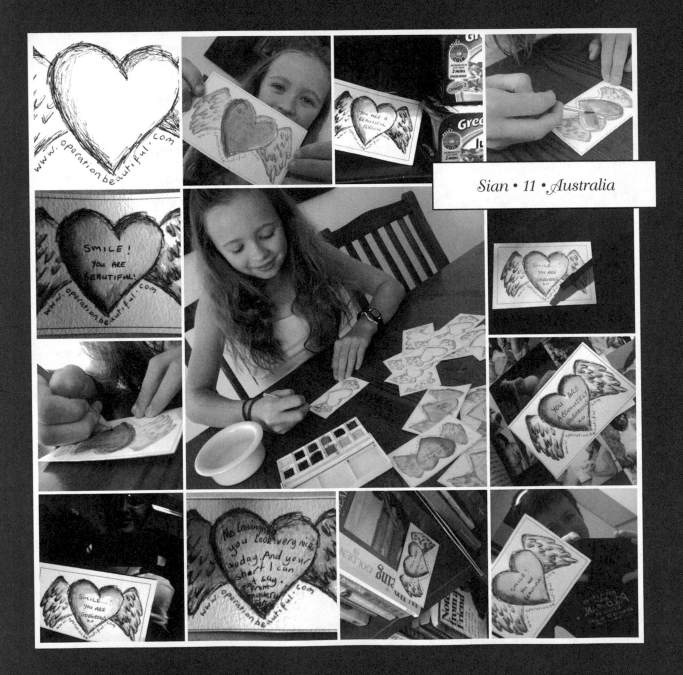

Sian • 11 • Australia

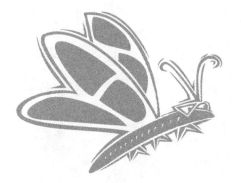

"I was having an extremely bad week. I had a twenty-page essay due on Wednesday and a ten-page essay due on Friday, both of which I had finished by Tuesday night and just had to read over once more Wednesday morning to catch any mistakes. I lost my USB port that night and had to redo both of them, on top of another ten-page report that was due the following Tuesday! I was extremely negative all week and generally in a horrible mood. I walked into a bathroom and there were Operation Beautiful Post-its with positive sayings all over one wall. The top Post-it said 'Take one.' On the mirror was a card that read, 'You look lovely today and every day. You are a beautiful woman' with the Operation Beautiful website on the bottom. I had never heard of this, but I thought it was wonderful. Seeing all the positive sayings on the wall really picked me up and made me smile. I took a note that said 'Healthy and Happy' to remind me to stay positive. Thank you for this experience!"

Lindsay Geisler • 21 • Saskatoon, Saskatchewan, Canada

"Making others happy is what truly makes me happy, especially during times when being happy is . . . pretty difficult. Mention money and many of us feel like oozing onto the ground. The economy is the ultimate Debbie Downer. I felt this while sitting in a bank's drive-through teller one day. I got to stressing about how I was going to pay for 'this' and if I would be able to afford 'that.' The thoughts were so overwhelming that I began to get pretty depressed. Then, I remembered the pre-written Operation Beautiful stickies I left in my purse. I put one on the chute, and it made me smile knowing that it would make the person behind me smile, too. It wouldn't instantly change our money situations but it would remind us to value something more than money: ourselves. And that's the thing about spreading positive messages: All parties involved benefit."

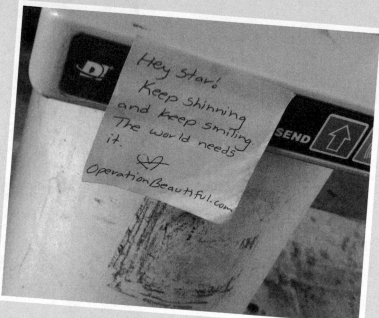

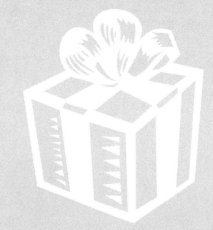

Brittany • 24 • Orlando, Florida

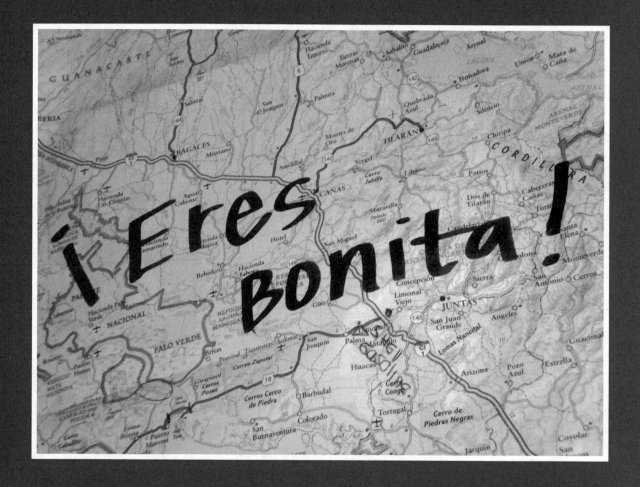

¡Eres Bonita!

"Ryan and I dated until he ended the relationship our junior year in college. I was devastated. Ryan was—and is—an amazing guy. He's smart, attractive, easygoing, and I have never met someone who made me laugh as loudly and as often as he could. If I couldn't make it work with a person like that, I thought to myself, the problem was in me. For a year after we broke up, I couldn't pass a mirror without scrutinizing every part of my appearance. I must have been too fat for him. My skin tone was too uneven. My legs were too stumpy. My breasts were too small. It was exhausting living this way.

I applied to, and was accepted by, a top-ten law school. The summer before my first year, I spent two months volunteering in Costa Rica at a women's environmentalist grassroots organization called AMURECI. The ladies at AMURECI operated a small store where they sold crafts to raise money and awareness for women's and environmental issues in their community. Every morning, each lady would greet me with a kiss and a *pura vida*. Their lovely children would float in and out throughout the day, while we toiled away at our jewelry-making and painting. With the very little Spanish I knew, we chatted about their lives. I realized how happy these women were. They weren't size twos and they never will be. They had very little money, but no matter how little they had, it was enough. They loved their lives and their families, and that love made them glow. I saw in the women at AMURECI that outer beauty is simply a manifestation of inner beauty.

So, I returned home to my loving family, who greeted me at the airport with 'Welcome Home!' posters and humongous hugs. I knew then it was okay that I

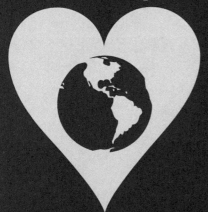 wasn't Kate Moss thin—who I am is enough. If Ryan no longer loved me, that was okay, too—what I had was enough. I have a family who loves me, a first-rate education, and a body that can do amazing things. And that is, and always will be, enough. I know that now."

Jane B. • 26 • Charlottesville, Virginia

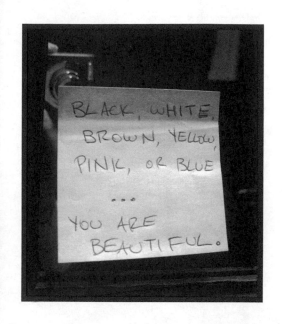

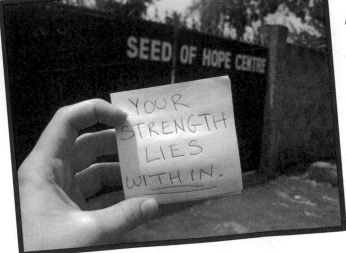

"*I posted the first note on a bathroom window in a coffeehouse in Nairobi, Kenya. Because Nairobi is a city defined by its wide range of ethnicities, I figured that a message of skin-color acceptance would be an appropriate sentiment. I posted the second on the front gate of the Seed of Hope Centre, which is a vocational, business, and life-skills training center that serves disadvantaged teenage girls from the slums of Nairobi. Some of the girls come from truly horrific situations: child marriage, prostitution, homelessness, and more. Although the Centre works to supply them with the tools to become self-sufficient and independent adults, I think it's important they remember that their drive to succeed ultimately comes from within.*"

Anna Chapin • 21 • Nairobi, Kenya

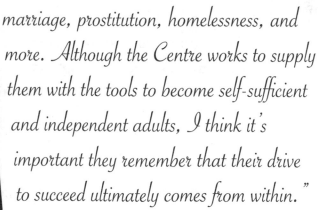

"I went on a trip from my home in Virginia to Pennsylvania and Delaware. On my way, I stuck a Post-it note with the message, 'You make the world a better place, just by being you!' on each of the bills I used to pay the toll operators. Each time I passed through a toll, I told the operator I wanted to pay for the person behind me, and I asked the toll operator to tell the people in these cars to have a beautiful day. I hope that the people receiving these gifts passed them on and paid for the cars behind them, too! Doing this made me feel as if my trip had a purpose—to help others and make them feel beautiful."

Ilene Gillispie • 19 • Florida

"I was walking through the Charlotte airport when I saw a blind man with a white cane doing the best he could to go from one gate to another. A young man asked him if he could walk with him to his gate. He said yes and mentioned that he travels a couple times a year and doesn't like to ask the airlines to assist him. He added that he never has any problem making it to his flight on time because some special person seems to always appear and he enjoys the stranger's genuine kindness. They walked away to his gate. I was so touched I posted this note on the airport's suggestion box."

Joy • 64 • Tennessee

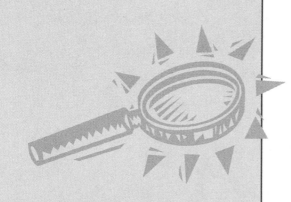

The Big Picture

It's a familiar scene on talk shows: A weepy woman who survived a traumatic event will say something like, "I never really appreciated my family/health/friend/life/freedom/job until it was almost taken away from me!" The host will thoughtfully nod and the audience will politely clap. As viewers, we think, "What a great lesson." Maybe we even shed a tear. But then a commercial comes on, and we change the channel without a second thought.

It is clichéd but so true: We often fail to focus on the things that really matter. Instead of treating ourselves with kindness and nurturing relationships with family and friends, we obsess over minute problems that simply don't matter in the grand scheme of life. Imagine how it would feel at the end of your life to look back and think, "I cherished every moment."

Here are some simple ways
to lead a more focused, appreciative life:

- Little miscommunications, hassles, mistakes, and annoyances serve to shift our focus from the pivotal to the trivial. How many hours have you wasted ruminating over your rude coworkers' behavior, your spiteful mother-in-law, or the stranger who cut you off on the freeway? When you feel yourself becoming upset over a small issue, take a deep breath and think, "What else could I do with this time and energy?" Whatever the issue, let it go.

- One technique for letting it go is to simply visualize the negative energy you feel building inside you as a hot, red ball of light. Imagine all your irritation flowing into the center of your body, into the red ball. Once you feel that the ball contains all your negative energy, visualize yourself pushing it away from the center of your body and it bouncing away.

- Similarly, it is important to choose your battles. Many people feel nitpicked by their partners; constantly pointing out another's faults or mistakes is hurtful and breeds resentment. Not even one can be—or should be—molded to fit your ideals and preferences. Learn to let some differences stand. Take a deep breath before you confront someone.

- Try not to rely on other people for your happiness. People are not perfect, and you set yourself up for disappointment if you depend on others to validate, uplift, and support you. This is not meant to imply that other people cannot enhance and enrich your life. Happiness is a boat—you are the hull, and other people are your sails. You may not go very fast without sails, but you cannot sink if the hull is intact.

- Practice being alone—go for a walk in the park or write in your journal—or challenge yourself to try something new without the assistance of a friend or significant other. The greatest gift you can give yourself is self-reliance. Put your relationship with yourself first.

- Accept this fact: Bad things happen to good people for no particular reason. Such is life. It is more than acceptable to wallow in your misery, to feel grief and pain, to express sadness for a moment. There must be a time when you think, "Enough is enough," and you choose to actively move forward. Be proactive in your recovery; do things that make you happy. Seek the assistance of a professional if you feel especially troubled.

- React with love. This is not a sign of weakness; it does not mean you are wrong or the other person is right. Reacting with love, understanding, and acceptance diffuses tense situations and prevents many arguments. When you feel a disagreement brewing, ask yourself, "How can I react with love right now?" It may be as simple as hugging the other person, listening without interrupting, or admitting that an opposing point is valid.

- When you react with love during an argument, the other person may initially be confused. The person may rebuff your loving gesture with suspicion. Reacting with love is not a one-shot deal; express it even when the other person cannot. Your reaction can be unconditional to his or her reaction. This does not mean you must engage people if they are being hostile; sometimes, reacting with love means simply walking away until you have calmed down.

- Reconcile the difference between what you want and what you need. So much unhappiness is created by pining for things we want but do not need— a bigger house, a better car, perfect clothes, smoother skin, more money, a slimmer figure. The greater the gap between what you want and what you need to survive, the more unhappy you will be. Instead of comparing yourself to people who have more things than you, compare yourself to the vast majority of the world and consider yourself lucky and blessed. Be thankful for all that you have.

A Bridge

The happiest people don't necessarily have *everything*—they might not have a "perfect" body, pretty clothes, or a nice car; they might not have a loving spouse or significant other; they might even struggle to pay the bills or have a serious health problem. True happiness requires just one thing: faith.

Initially, some people balk at the word "faith," as it is often identified with organized religion. The religious certainly have faith in their beliefs, but faith can also exist without religion. Faith does not necessitate prayer or pews. There are many different kinds of faith: faith that tomorrow will be better than today, faith in the power of love, faith in the intrinsic goodness of others, faith that a missed opportunity was never meant to be, faith that life is more than a series of random occurrences, faith in yourself.

Faith is a bridge to contentment. It is as integral to being happy and healthy as eating a balanced diet; faith is as important as staying active. You can gnaw on carrot sticks and do sit-ups all day long, but you'll never find contentment if you cannot look around this crazy, mixed-up world we live in and see purpose in some small way. Your own unique brand of faith will carry you through the ho-hum of everyday life and comfort you when you're challenged mentally, emotionally, and physically.

Heather Shugarman never saw it coming. She had

spent the weekend away with her bridesmaids and friends, making final plans for her wedding, which was six weeks away. Her fiancé picked her up from the airport and drove her to her apartment, chatting like everything was fine. The wedding invitations were dropped in the mail the next day. "I had just returned home when my fiancé called to say he was stopping by," she remembers. "He came over, and I was so excited to talk about all the wedding 'to do's' I had gotten done." But he stopped her mid-sentence and dropped the bomb: He could not marry her. The wedding was off.

"I felt so many different emotions at the same time—so sad, heartbroken, hurt, humiliated, angry, sarcastic, a bit sick, in denial, and somewhat happy that he told me now and not later," Heather says. "I fell into a bit of an emotional pit. I questioned my worth and my identity. Deep down in my heart, I knew I was good enough. I knew I was beautiful. I knew I was worthy of love and life and success and joy. But some days, it was a struggle to remember these things. Some days, I was just numb."

Heather decided to redefine herself. After being part of a couple for so long, many people in her life didn't know Heather for Heather—she was just someone's girlfriend. She set out to shake up some aspects of her life, starting with a drastic haircut that made her feel fabulous. Her quest to be healthier, which had begun before the breakup, was renewed. "I decided that the bad in my life was not going to win," she says.

A few weeks later, Heather took a road trip and met a friend in a city neither had ever been to before. They visited a museum and posted Operation Beautiful notes all over the displays in the children's wing. "On my drive back home, I

started thinking about the truth that was in our notes, and how grateful I was to have posted it. And I could feel my heart beginning to heal a bit," Heather says. She continued to post notes, sticking kind messages almost everywhere she went. "I posted notes in bathrooms. I handed notes to toll booth operators. I left notes on car doors," she says. One day at the bookstore, she spent "a few hours strategically placing notes of truth and worth in books and nooks and shelves and magazines."

For Heather, her intense participation in Operation Beautiful was an extension of the faith she already had in her heart, a belief that was there before she met her fiancé, deepened as they worked together at their church, and matured after the breakup. Heather's faith is rooted in her religious choices. "One of my New Year's resolutions before we got together was to spend twelve hours being silent. And so I took off a random Wednesday in early January and sat at my house. I read the Bible and other books. I journaled and I prayed. I sat on my porch and listened to birds," she says. "And I read a passage in Ephesians that made an analogy between being a child and being a Christian. That a baby doesn't drink milk forever, eventually he has to eat solid food for nourishment. As a Christian, what we first use to sustain our relationship with Christ isn't enough forever. We need something more 'solid.' And it hit me hard. What was I doing now that was different than before? Where could I go deeper? Where could I get more *sustenance*? I prayed and meditated on the word. And felt like I should volunteer my time."

Heather began to dedicate much of her free time to a group of teenage girls at her church, leading discussion groups and one-on-one mentoring dates. "I love showing them they are loved, and unique, and beautiful. Teaching them how to stand tall and be proud of who they are. And the moment you see them realize, admit, know, or believe that they are wonderful, beautiful creatures that are deserving of their hearts' desires . . . that is enough right then to give you faith," she observes. "They ministered to me so much more than I could have ever ministered to them."

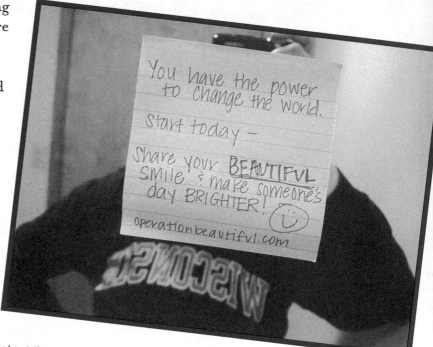

Other people might have crumbled under the pressure of the breakup, but Heather refused to turn inward and ruminate on the marriage that never was. Instead, she drew on the strength gained from mentoring the girls at church and posting Operation Beautiful notes for strangers. "Faith is the choice that I made," she says. Her faith assured her that there was purpose in her heartbreak, and helping others allowed her to heal herself.

Heather Shugarman • 26 • Scotia, New York

"I believe that if you surround yourself with the positive, there will be no room for negative," she says. "I love that when I write 'You are beautiful' on a note to leave behind for total strangers, I begin to believe it myself. I love that when I take the time to encourage others, I find myself encouraged."

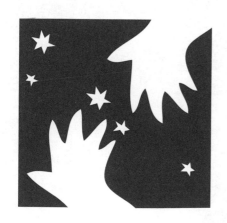

"I was buying fabric to make eighteen napkins for a luncheon for the nurses at the neonatal intensive care unit. There was a short, very heavy woman in her fifties behind the fabric counter. Her face was a little distorted, and her tongue was kind of 'thick' and odd. She could hardly stand up and had to hold on as she walked around the counter.

I think of myself as generally nonjudg-mental when it comes to how people look, but I noticed that I had made the judgment that she probably wasn't very smart, and I should make sure she measured my fabric correctly. Then I thought to myself, 'This is not beau-tiful thinking, Beth. Be more open and kind to her.' Well, as I was thinking this she asked me what I was making. I told her, and she en-gaged me in a conversation about why I needed so many napkins, and how pretty they would be, and how wonderful nurses are, and that the napkins would also look great with a red tablecloth. She was an absolute delight to talk to. The nicest ten minutes I had all day.

It was such a good lesson. I think that if I had not changed my thinking toward her, I would not have been able to respond to her. The other thing I thought was that she must see herself as beautiful and be comfortable with who she is to engage a stranger in such a warm conversation. I'm wondering if she sensed my anxiety over all I had to get done for the luncheon and was trying to help ME! It was a really meaningful experience."

Beth Talaga • 56 • Gainesville, Florida

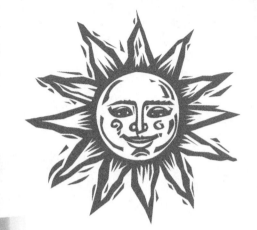

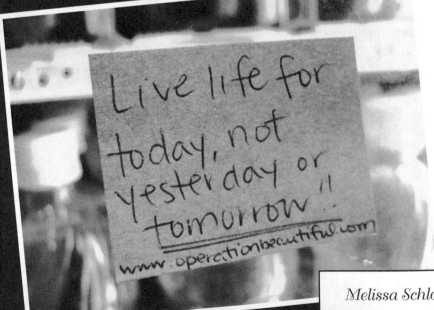

Live life for today, not yesterday or tomorrow!!

www.operationbeautiful.com

Melissa Schlothan • 24 • California

232

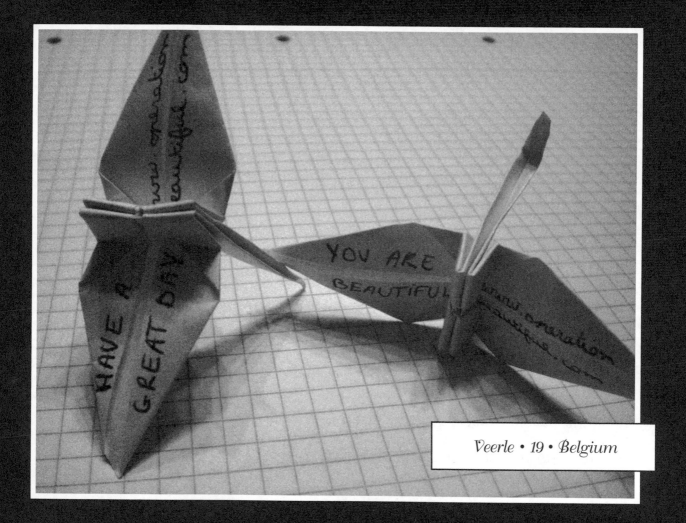

Veerle • 19 • Belgium

"During breaks at school, dull moments in class, on the bus home, or before I go to sleep, I fold some origami birds and write an Operation Beautiful message on each one. I leave the birds in the hallways or on my chair as I leave or on the bus. I do this in the hope that it could be the right message for the right person at the right time."

"Ever since first grade, I've wanted to be a teacher. The road to achieve this goal has been very bumpy, but I've always told myself that hard work pays off. I am now on my third year teaching at my high school alma mater. Because I am a product of this school, I am passionate about this community and feel that I have an obligation to make a positive impact on the school and my students. I recently had a very rough and disappointing day with a particular period. I felt like my efforts were not paying off in terms of motivating the students and helping them realize that good grades, graduating from high school, and thinking about college are directly related to success. I went home feeling hopeless.

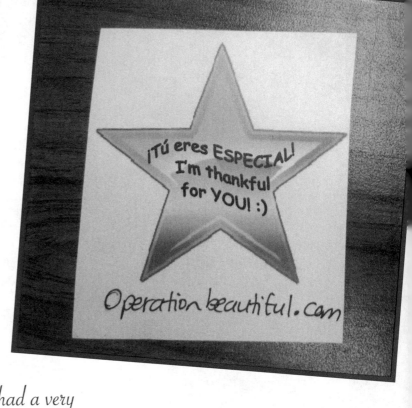

The next day, during my fourth-period class, a former student walked in and gave me a yellow piece of paper that said, 'You make someone out there smile. (Yes, YOU!) Keep your shining smile on display for the world to embrace. www.operationbeautiful.com.' I looked at her and smiled, a bit confused. She said, 'Thank you, Ms. Garcia. You have done a lot, really.' I admit my eyes got watery because I felt like it was the answer I was looking for the day before. That simple note refueled my hope and got me back on my feet in a second. My students were eager to know what it said, so I read it out loud and asked them if they knew what Operation Beautiful was. Nobody knew! I ran to the computer and typed it in. That is how I found out about its admirable mission.

I decided to create two hundred stars for my students and friends that said '¡Tú eres ESPECIAL! I'm thankful for you!' The next day, I placed a star on each desk. My students' reactions were priceless. Some said thank you, others simply smiled, and a few of them asked for a second star to give to a friend. Their sincere gratitude and smiles were the best gifts I have received in three years as a teacher."

Susana Garcia • 26 • Anaheim, California

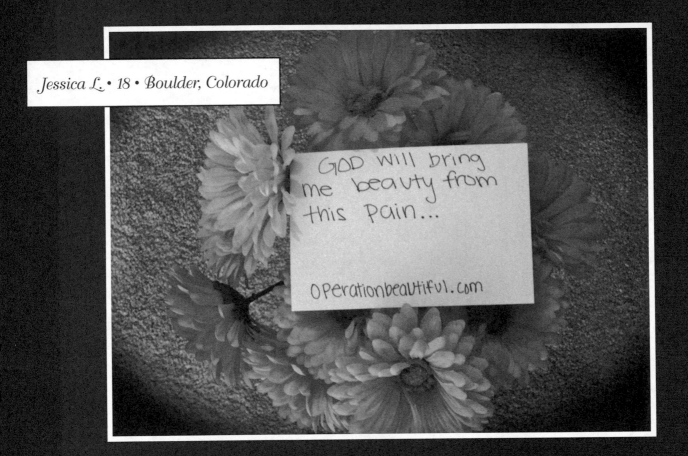

Jessica L. • 18 • Boulder, Colorado

GOD will bring me beauty from this pain...

OperationBeautiful.com

"I have always believed that God does things for a reason. But when someone experiences a tragedy, his or her image of God can be destroyed. Unfortunately, I experienced a terrible tragedy. When I was fourteen, I went away to boarding school and was repeatedly raped and molested for three months. For the past three years, I have been battling whether or not there is a God. Well, through music and my own intuition, I have come to the conclusion that God does exist. He thankfully got me out of boarding school and I do believe that one day, God will bring something beautiful from all of my pain and suffering."

"I posted this note on the mirror in McDonald's. I had seen a woman in the eating area that seemed to be closing in on herself. She looked like she had been crying. I remembered my Post-its in my purse, and I rushed off to the bathroom. I put the note on the mirror in the hope that it would brighten someone's day. Operation Beautiful really does help women. It is so important for us to feel amazing."

Lu • 33 • San Antonio, Texas

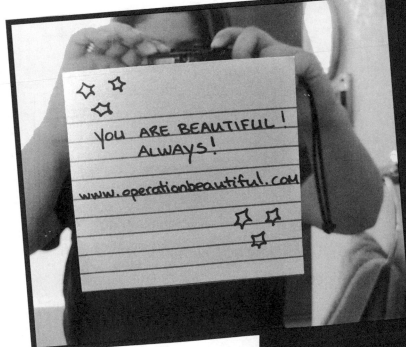

The Living Bible

Look at the reflection in your Creator's eyes to see your true beauty.

operationbeautiful.com

Andra K. • 12 • *Cleveland, Ohio*

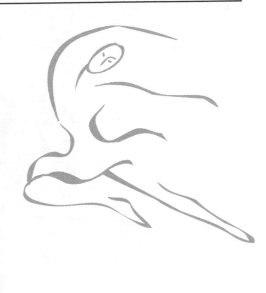

Gillian • 22 • *Paris, France*

"When I face my fears and do what I really want to, I feel beautiful. After graduating from university I decided to fly back to Paris, where I am now, attempting to write my first book. I may be terrified, broke, lonely, and drinking too many espressos, but I am so proud of myself. I am taking a chance because I believe in myself. That is beautiful."

You are beautiful
when you follow
your dreams

www.operation.beautiful.com

FINDING FAITH

It might seem easier to be cynical. A tough attitude seems like an impermeable suit of armor, protecting us from expecting too much and getting hurt. But pessimism also hardens us until we feel hollow and empty inside. Our jaded outlook becomes a self-fulfilling prophecy; it results in so many missed opportunities and failed dreams. We begin to believe that happiness is something that happens to other people. We're left with the inability to love and trust.

Faith softens us and fills that hollow spot with hope. Even if you are not optimistic by nature, you can change your attitude and approach to life. It is possible to become a more hopeful person, and the results of your attitude change may surprise you.

Having faith is not necessarily about being religious. You can create your own type of faith based on your trust in others, hope for a better tomorrow, belief in a higher power, or love for the miracle of everyday life.

Here are simple exercises for finding your faith:

- How many times have you thought, "Tomorrow, I will finally go to the gym," "Tomorrow, I will call

my old best friend," or "Tomorrow, I will volunteer for a charity"? The root of this procrastination is fear. We may think things like, "It doesn't matter what I do. My situation will never get better." We live our lives trapped by the fear of disappointment, failure, and rejection.

- Many people spend years—even a lifetime—fixating on a single slight or a broken promise. They may ruminate over disasters they cannot prevent or control. After years of thinking like this, a person becomes spiritually depleted. Their bodies may rebel under the emotional stress and become more susceptible to chronic ailments such as heart disease and cancer. Years of negative thinking can make it challenging to integrate present living into your daily life.

- You must train yourself to have faith and live for today; otherwise, you may find yourself paralyzed with the obsession over yesterday and tomorrow. Present living does not mean you ignore life lessons or stop planning for the future; however, it does allow you to stop treating life like one giant emergency. Present living requires you to ask yourself, "Is this really a big deal?" and "Should I really be getting upset and negative over this?"

- When you are experiencing a happy moment, pause and take it all in. Too often we think, "Ah, this is nice!" and then move on to the next task. Take deep breaths and try to remember the moment with all of your five senses. The next time you find yourself living outside of the present, remember your last happy moment and try to capture the peacefulness you felt at that time.

- When you feel lost, fearful, or anxious, remind yourself that you cannot control others' actions or be held responsible for others' emotions. Identify what aspects of the situation you have the power to change, if any, and take action to improve your mental attitude. Ask yourself if you've ever encountered a similar situation; in hindsight, should you have approached the experience in a different way? How can you apply the lessons of your past to today?

- Consider the possibility that everything happens for a reason. This does not imply an absence of free will or that the order of your life is predetermined by a higher power. It is simply a confidence that each experience, no matter how exciting, disappointing, sad, or joyous, is propelling you toward a bigger purpose.

- If the idea that everything has a purpose sounds too far-out for you, try this exercise. Consider your present situation and the complex path that led you to this point. For example, perhaps you love your

job, and you never would have been hired if you hadn't completed an internship with the company while you were in college. Maybe you would've never interned at that specific company if your best friend forgot to tell you about the opportunity. You wouldn't even know your best friend if you had sat in a different seat on the first day of class. You might not have attended that specific college without the scholarship you received, and perhaps you would not have gotten the scholarship without writing a powerful essay on growing up with an alcoholic parent. Although your childhood was terribly rough, you owe many of the good things—your college education, friendships, job—to the path that it put you on.

- The belief that your life is not random and that each experience is a learning opportunity is quite freeing. When we are confronted with a challenge, this belief frees us from the troubling "What if?" or "Why me?" cycle. Instead of obsessing about past mistakes or future scenarios, we can focus on the present and trust that the current challenge serves a larger purpose.

- Have you ever watched a particularly cheerful and charismatic person walk into a room? The whole crowd turns, captivated by their positive, joyful energy. Similarly, a person who feels extremely low or angry brings the mood of others down, too.

Now, take this concept one step further—each cell in our bodies is alive with this energy. Your whole body radiates either positive or negative energy to the people you interact with, which impacts their energy.

Some people have faith that "good things happen to good people" or "you reap what you sow." These beliefs are based upon the observation that you can use your energy—or, more concretely, your time and attention—to create goodness in your own life and in the lives of others. Believe in your own power to create happiness in your life. You have the power to take any situation and put a positive, optimistic spin on it. You have the power to react with kindness and understanding. You have the power to live in the present. Life doesn't happen to you; make life happen for you.

• Perhaps the simplest—and most profound—way to gain your own kind of faith is to realize you are not alone. We are all human; we are all struggling with the same day-to-day achievements and letdowns. This principle is what Operation Beautiful was founded on. Even when we feel hopeless, tired, ugly, or sad, we can reach out to a stranger through an anonymous message. We can transmit our energy of goodwill to others and receive a dose in return, all through a little piece of paper.

Chapter 7

Going Forward

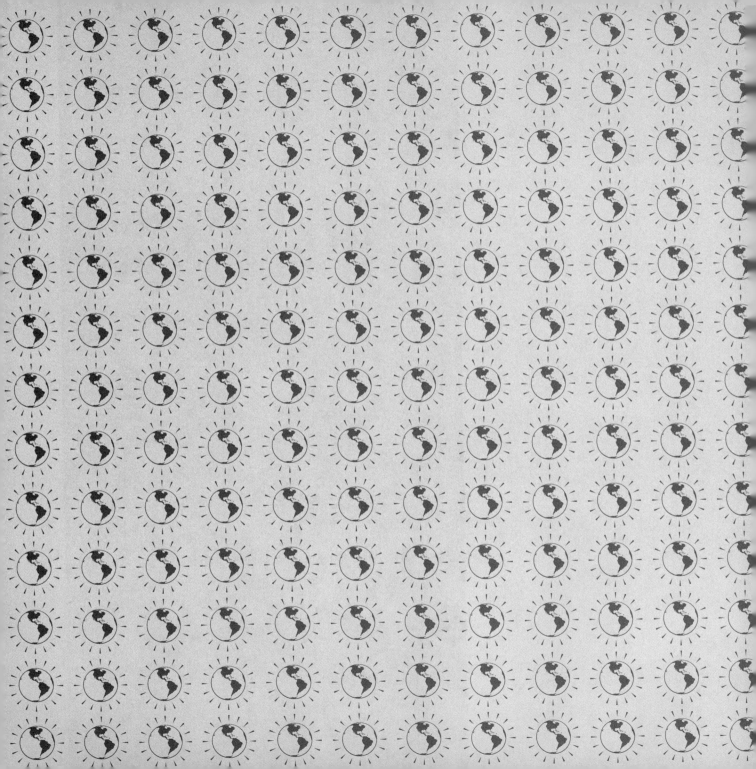

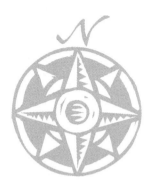

Going Forward

*M*y name is Caitlin, and I am learning.

Many years ago, I resisted my own need to grow and discover. Looking inward with a critical eye is a hard—and sometimes painful—process. I sensed there was an emotional and spiritual journey inside my own heart, but I feared asking myself the hard questions. Not starting the conversation at all was much easier. I focused on small, unimportant things to distract me from the issues that really mattered. I got caught up in trivial arguments; I Fat Talked; I stayed on the couch instead of living my life.

Meanwhile, the questions continued to sound in my heart. Who am I? What do I really want? *What am I so afraid of?*

I was scared of examining myself. Admitting that I was powerful enough to change my life, but was simply too lazy or apathetic, was frightening. This very thought put all the responsibility on my own shoulders and was

My beauty comes from my willingness to learn.

overwhelming—I would no longer be able to blame rotten luck, other people, or my love of cookies for my unhappiness.

Operation Beautiful was the last piece of the puzzle for me. With one Post-it, I unlocked the secret to my own empowerment. Operation Beautiful took away my fear, and as I peeled back my emotional defenses, I saw myself for who I really was—and it was beautiful. I realized I was capable of changing my life for the better. I deserved it. I now understand that there is always room for personal growth, but I never needed to "fix" any part of me. I realized that it's okay not to be perfect. I make plenty of mistakes in my life. I overdraw my bank account; I pick fights with my husband about the dirty laundry; I never change the oil in my car; I accidentally say hurtful things; I forget to return library books for months on end; I'd rather eat a big bowl of ice cream instead of vegetables. I make mistakes, and life goes on.

My beauty has nothing to do with perfection. My beauty comes from my willingness to learn. I was afraid of this journey because I wasn't sure where it would end, but now I realize that there is no end. To truly live my life, I must be always growing, failing, succeeding, changing, *learning*.

In some curious way, spreading love to other people through anonymous notes helped me learn to love myself. After all, if I could acknowledge and embrace the imperfections in strangers, how could I not look inward and do the same for myself? I truly believe in the power of positivity and random acts of kindness. These actions show us who we are and what we are capable of achieving.

It is my sincerest hope that Operation Beautiful will assist you as you travel down your own path to self-love and acceptance.

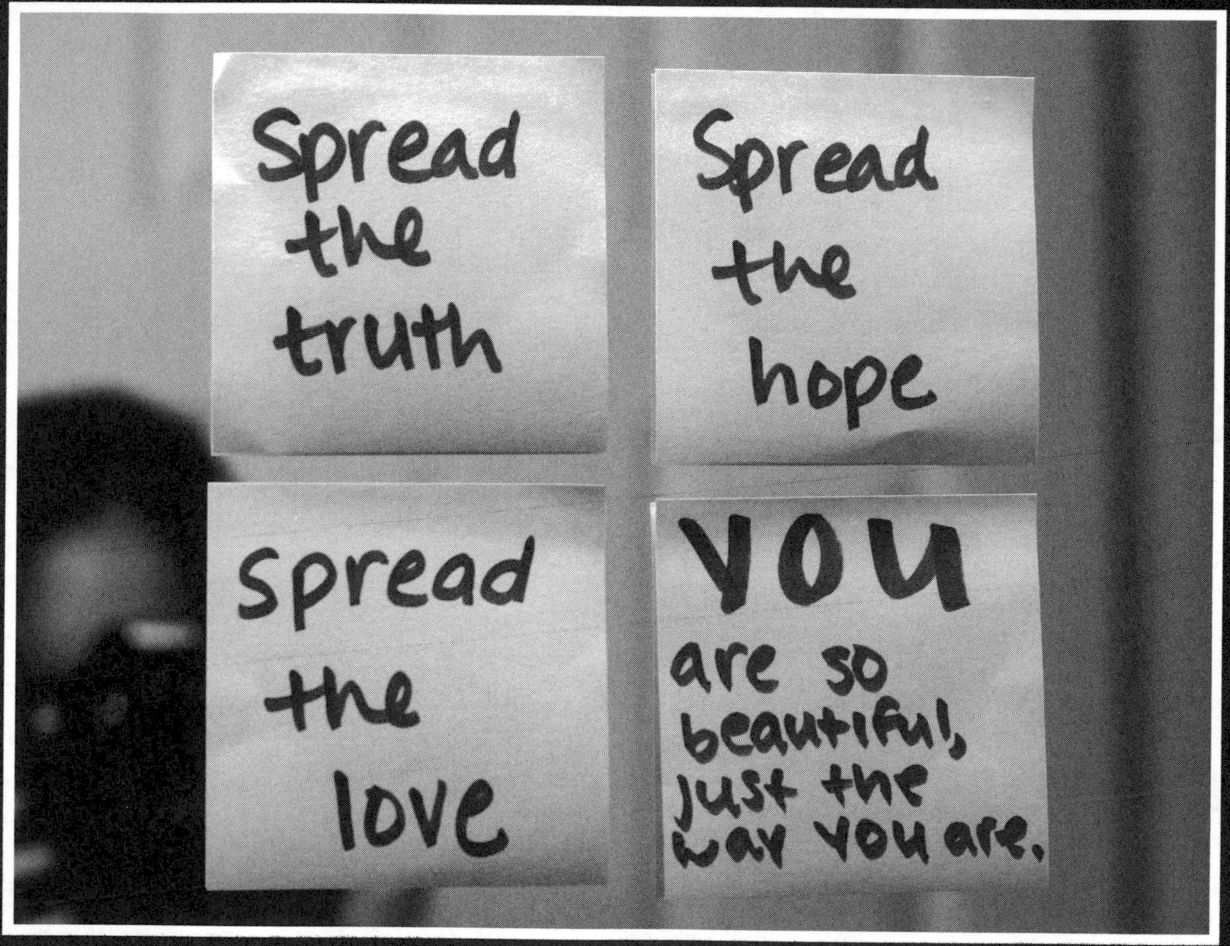
Spread the truth
Spread the hope
Spread the love
YOU are so beautiful, just the way you are.

MOTIVATIONAL MANTRAS

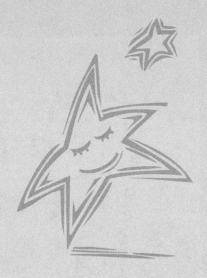

There's nothing better than a great quote to inspire and uplift. Here are a list of Operation Beautiful's favorite motivational mantras—repeat these to yourself when you need a boost or write the messages on a note for a stranger to find!

- Stop waiting for the "perfect moment" to begin your life because it will never come. Embrace your life today!

- When the world says, "Give up," hope whispers, "Give it one more try." Believe in yourself, and you can achieve any goal.

- Love isn't love until you give it away.

- What will be, will be. It will all work out.

- Don't pray for a lighter load; pray for a stronger back.

- Expect things to be perfect, and you will drown in the ebb and flow of life. Pessimists hold themselves back from succeeding. Find the opportunities in difficulties and new potentials in failures.

- You have the power to refocus your time and energy on things that really matter. You have the willpower to let the small things slide.

- There is always tomorrow.

- You are enough, just the way you are!

- One day at a time; one foot in front of the other.

- Your power is beyond your comprehension. You can do anything.

- If you want to transform your life, dig deep down and find the commitment to change. Change does not come from other people or things. The power to grow into who you want to be is already inside of you.

- You are transforming into who you want to become. You are transformed.

- Life is an adventure!

- The only thing standing between you and your goal is yourself and your fear. Be fearless!

- Everything will be okay in the end, and if it's not okay, it's not the end.

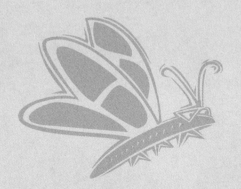

- Count your blessings whenever you feel down—you have so much to be grateful for!

- You're only worth what you sell yourself for. Don't sell yourself short—you're priceless.

- The key to success is not to set any limits. You can do it!

- Live in the present. The troubles of tomorrow and the uncertainties of the future have no control over you.

- What are your dreams? It is impossible to achieve what you don't acknowledge. Dream big!

- You are so much stronger than you think you are.

- To be upset over what you do not have is to waste all the things you are blessed with.

- Happiness is a choice.

- Limited expectations yield limited results.

- Find beauty in the things you see every day—including yourself.

- Take time to cherish yourself—you are worth it!

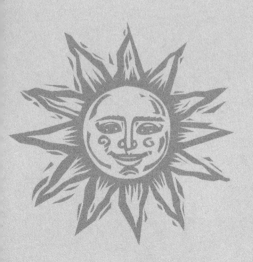

- Life doesn't happen to you; make life happen for you.

- Commit to living openly, truthfully, and freely. Be your authentic self.

- Challenges bring opportunities. Embrace it, and you will thrive!

- Be the best version of yourself today!

- Hello, Masterpiece!

- Everything is getting better every day. Believe it, and it is so.

- The most amazing surprises are uncovered when you blaze your own trail.

- Pessimism and optimism are self-fulfilling prophecies. Your situation should not determine your attitude. Your attitude determines your situation. Choose to be happy and hopeful. Choose optimism!

- You already have everything you need.

- Change the way you see, not the way you look.

- Nothing is more powerful than hope.

- I've never seen a smiling face that was not beautiful.

- Beauty comes in all shapes, sizes, and ages because true beauty shines from the inside out.

- Look at the wonder that is your body, your brain, your being. You are a miracle!

- Self-compassion is the first step out of whatever difficulty we're in.

- Yesterday is history, tomorrow is a mystery, but today is a gift. That's why they call it the present.

- You're never given more than you can handle. You are strong enough to overcome any obstacle and thrive in all situations.

- Know that there is nothing you cannot accomplish. When you doubt yourself, draw on your past triumphs over hard adversity.

- Your imperfections make you unique.

Acknowledgments

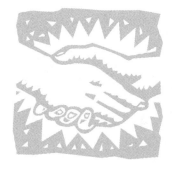

*M*any thanks are owed to the girls, women, and men who read the Operation Beautiful blog on a daily basis. You made Operation Beautiful into the international movement it is today. Thank you for spreading the love and changing countless lives!

To the more than two hundred women who shared their stories for the *Operation Beautiful* book—thank you. Your strength and determination to be the best version of yourself are so admirable, and I learned a great deal interviewing each one of you. Thank you for giving a bit of yourself to this book.

I'd also like to acknowledge the wonderful, inspiring, and thought-provoking food and fitness blog community. My life would be so different without your support and friendship. A special thanks is owed to Katy Widrick, my media-savvy friend who had the smarts to tell our local paper about Operation Beautiful.

Thanks to the professionals who contributed their wisdom to this book. Your knowledge was invaluable and shaped this book into a tool that people can use to better their own lives.

Thanks to the crew at Gotham Books, especially Miriam Rich, for helping transform *Operation Beautiful* into such a wonderful book. And last—but certainly not least—I owe so much to Chris Park, my agent at Foundry Literary + Media who started me on this amazing journey. Thank you for believing in *Operation Beautiful* from the start.

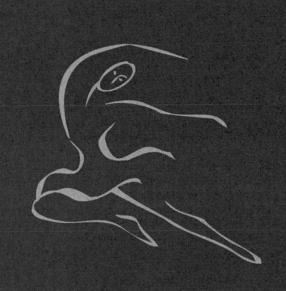

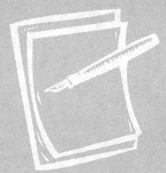

You are Beautiful!